Pain Free With Far Infrared Mineral Therapy

Pain Free With Far Infrared Mineral Therapy

The Miracle Lamp

Kara Lee Schoonover

iUniverse, Inc.
New York Lincoln Shanghai

Pain Free With Far Infrared Mineral Therapy
The Miracle Lamp

iUniverse, Inc.

For information address:
iUniverse, Inc.
2021 Pine Lake Road, Suite 100
Lincoln, NE 68512
www.iuniverse.com

The information contained in this book is not to be construed as medical advice.   It is my account of personal experiences, interpretation, and understanding of the far infrared mineral lamp or TDP lamp.

ISBN: 0-595-27263-0

Printed in the United States of America

*This book is dedicated to Muffin, my beloved canine friend, and all my two-legged friends desiring to be pain free **without** the use of harmful and many times ineffective drugs.*

Contents

Acknowledgments

I would like to thank Tano Lucero, Oriental Medical Doctor (OMD), for introducing me to the far infrared mineral lamp, his teachings, and his influence to take responsibility for my health care. I was so surprised when he invited me (a non-medical person) to register for one of his educational seminars, as my perception was that only professional medical personnel were entitled to learn new health care techniques. As the new me developed, I realized how valuable the far infrared mineral lamp could be in my home—it would give me more self-reliance and greatly reduce and/or eliminate the need for expensive doctor bills and harmful drugs.

Foreword

By Dr. Jing Yang Na

Traditional trained Chinese medical doctors have used the far infrared mineral lamp successfully. This lamp is great for various medical conditions and has been used in many hospitals all over China for several decades. It is popular with acupuncturist, surgical physicians, and physical therapy departments in the Chinese hospitals.

Because of its apparent results for pain relief and other benefits, it is also known as the "magic lamp." As a Chinese Doctor, I am happy that Kara has written a book about her personal experiences of using the infrared mineral lamp or "magic lamp."

As both a patient and a user, Kara has done an excellent job in sharing and explaining the use of the lamp and how it works, what it is good for, and how to use it. She has a lot of personal experiences and has done extensive study about the infrared mineral lamp. I found it interesting to see the difference in what the American users think of this lamp and how they explain the lamp.

This book is very beneficial to both users and health professionals alike. Enjoy the information Kara shares in this wonderfully written book of knowledge!

Dr. Jing Yang Na
Healing Arts Clinic by the River
Maple Valley, Washington

xi

Preface

While employed as a safety director and return-to-work program administrator in a small manufacturing company, I became aware of the ineffectiveness of drugs and surgery in relieving work-related soft tissue injuries and other health issues occurring in an office and manufacturing environment. I received education and training on work-related health problems through seminars sponsored by the Department of Labor and Industries and private companies who develop and market products that help in the reduction and elimination of some of these problems. It was my responsibility to research and implement alternatives that would reduce the risk of these employee work-related problems.

While our traditional medical doctors can provide the finest technology in the world in treating emergency-type problems, I believe that alternative therapies such as the far infrared mineral lamp are far superior in the treatment of soft tissue injuries and stress related health problems. Tendonitis, carpal tunnel, strains, and sprains are painful conditions that are difficult to heal on a permanent basis using drugs and surgery, yet they are a risk associated with jobs that require repetitive movement from employees. Overuse is the most common cause of tendonitis, which is characterized by chronic inflammation, tissue degeneration, and cell atrophy. Many employees are released for work with pain as a constant companion and/or forced to look for other types of employment because drug therapy has been ineffective in reducing the pain. The only other alternative offered by Western medicine is surgery, which too often only worsens the condition.

One of the benefits sometimes associated with the far infrared mineral lamp is light therapy. Lack of full-spectrum lighting in the office environment can also create work-related health problems. Cool-white fluorescent lighting is believed to increase hyperactivity, fatigue, and irritability. The effects of sunlight are similar to physical exercise since sunlight can increase the oxygen level in cells, muscle strength, and vitality. Sunlight can provide mental stability as evidenced in the Northwest by the increase in depression during the rainy season. It is believed that sunlight helps regulate hormonal activity, enhance immune function, and facilitate bone growth.

I believe the far infrared mineral lamp provides the most effective pain relief, anti-aging, and light therapy available today and a closely kept secret from many Americans suffering with pain, depression, fatigue, and premature aging.

Introduction

The senior market is the fastest growing segment of our population. Currently seniors are purported to control seventy-five percent of the wealth in the United States, and the sixty-five plus age group is the largest segment of the population. I recently read that current statistics indicate eighty percent of seniors have degenerative medical conditions that include osteoporosis, arthritis, heart disease, digestive disorders, diabetes, hypertension and cancer. It is my understanding that Medicare, the government's financially troubled program, covers drugs administered in hospitals, doctor's offices, and clinics for almost forty million elderly and disabled Americans, but does not cover outpatient prescription drugs. Prescription drug coverage was a big issue in the 2002 election campaign as a result of Congress failing to agree on a national Medicare plan. According to an article published in the one of the national newspapers, prices of the prescription drugs most commonly used by senior citizens rose nearly three times the inflation rate in 2001.

I am sixty-four years old and do not use prescription drugs, over-the-counter drugs, or street drugs of any kind. How is this possible? For starters, I see health care professionals that provide a level of care that takes the entire person into account. Proper nutrition, clean air, unpolluted water, and exercise greatly boosts my immune system. In addition, I use far infrared mineral lamp therapy, a powerful and effective alternative health remedy without the painful side effects of drugs or surgery.

Bothered with knee joint pain, tendonitis, stomach disorders, and a myriad of other aches and pains associated with the aging process, I was faced with the prospect of eventually succumbing to drugs and/or major surgery and had become one of several million Americans (some estimate one is every seven) suffering from inflamed, enlarged, and swollen joints, and loss of flexibility of the ligaments and muscles surrounding the joints. Some people have estimated arthritic complaints of which rheumatoid and osteoarthritis are the most common, affect the economy to the extent of billions of dollars in medicine and lost income annually.

Conventional (allopathic) medicine considers arthritis incurable but manageable. Some of the standard conventional treatments are a combination of medica-

1

tions, exercise, rest, hydrotherapy, and surgery. Anti-inflammatory drugs that temporarily stop the pain can have side effects such as upset stomach and ulcers. As the diseases progresses, cortisone and steroid injections are sometimes given with a risk of more serious side effects. A couple of years ago I was unaware that I was using a fraudulent anti-aging remedy prescribed by my medical doctor that contained a high amount of a cortisone-type medication. Upon discontinuance of the drug my naturopathic doctor treated me for severe adrenal suppression and other complications resulting from prolonged use of the drug.

The far infrared mineral lamp is unique in that the FDA has approved it for use by the general public in treating pain. The Chinese have successfully used it on millions of people with over a hundred different diseases and health problems. These clinical studies have shown the lamp to decrease inflammation and edema from soft tissue injuries such as strains, sprains, relieve arthritic pain, promote circulation and healing, balance the nervous system, and repair skin problems with no harmful side effects.

The far infrared mineral lamp has a very study three-legged stand with rollers. It is lightweight, easy to move and dismantle when traveling, and takes approximately five minutes to warm up. This unique device has a timer, and I often fall asleep while using it because the heat feels goods and is relaxing.

I am very thankful to the Chinese for this modern technology and its availability to lay people like myself.

1

The Lamp With a Crooked Neck

I was apprehensive! I had never been to an Oriental Medical Doctor (OMD) before and was uncomfortable lying on a massage table under a sheet, waiting for him to join me in the treatment room. The light in the room was dim, and in the dark shadows of the room I saw something that reminded me of a snake or maybe it was E.T., the lovable movie alien, staring at me. The object was in an upright position with a very crooked neck and seemed to have several small eyes of different colors. After staring at the image for several minutes, I experienced a floating sensation and feared the object might have some kind of power that was pulling me towards it.

Fear and panic overwhelmed me! I tried to cling to the empty air surrounding me. Wishing to control my imagination, I recalled the concentration techniques that I had learned and used in natural childbirth and decided to occupy my mind with other thoughts in order to replace the panic and fear I was feeling.

My reflections took me back to when I first learned about this body worker. My massage therapist had introduced him to me and encouraged me to research his treatment program. Shortly thereafter, I attended a seminar he gave at a local health clinic and was surprised to learn that he was of Spanish descent, not Chinese. The information presented at the seminar revealed that the term, Oriental medical doctor, did not refer to his nationality but to the kind of medicine he practiced. He told us he was a Qigong practitioner and chose Traditional Chinese Medicine (TCM) to treat clients because of its many years of successful therapies.

My interpretation of what he said was that Chinese medicine is an ancient medical system (originating before Christ) and based on the view of a universe in which everything in interrelated and designed to promote and maintain health through diet and exercise (some principles of Qigong). Illnesses are treated with acupuncture, herbs, and energy exercises. Chinese medicine practitioners view the mind and body as an energetic system that cannot be separated from any of its parts or the universe. Organs are viewed as interconnected systems working together to keep the body working properly. Chinese medicine practitioners treat the whole patient, not the illness. An organ may be perceived as normal and healthy by Western medicine and be perceived as deficient by a TCM doctor.

The Chinese Way to Healing: Many Paths to Wholeness by Misha Ruth Cohen gives a great account of Chinese healing practices. The author gives direction and guidance in combining Chinese dietary guidelines and healing therapies with Western medicine in the treatment of a wide range of illnesses including stress, anxiety, depression, and digestive problems. This is a great book for people like myself who are interested in self-therapy and alternatives to drugs and surgery.

My thoughts reflected on my friend, Becky, who applied for and received social security disability payments at the age of fifty.

In earlier years, she had developed a malignant growth on her thyroid—the doctors performed a thyroidectomy. This is a procedure where the patient is given a general anesthetic; an incision is made in the front of the neck, and up to ninety percent of the gland surgically removed. The thyroid gland is part of the endocrine (hormone) system and plays a major role in regulating metabolism. Endocrine glands produce and secrete hormones into the blood or lymph system that may affect one organ or tissue or sometimes the entire body. The thyroid gland is found under the Adam's apple in the front part of the neck. It cannot be seen or felt in most people. It consists of two lobes united by a narrow isthmus.

The gland retrieves iodine from the blood absorbed from foods eaten to make the thyroid hormone required in many body functions. Most tumors that develop in the thyroid gland are benign or non-cancerous and sometimes appear as bumps in the neck. The surgical removal of her thyroid necessitated oral thyroid supplementation probably for the rest of her life. Thyroid cancers grow slowly and can recur years after treatment. Follow-up care continues for twenty to thirty years and may include blood tests, X-rays, and CT scans.

I believe a TCM doctor would have identified and corrected the imbalances in Beck's body years much earlier with acupuncture, herbs, and other natural remedies years before the cancerous tumor developed!

Becky told me she suffered with painful menstruation for many years. She felt that a woman's body deteriorates more rapidly after childbirth. To treat pain and other discomforts, the doctors performed a partial hysterectomy to relieve the pelvic pain and difficult menstrual periods. Removal of her uterus ended menstruation, her ability to become pregnant, and necessitated the use of oral estrogen therapy thereafter.

Becky told me there were numerous other surgeries throughout her adult life—each surgery relieving a specific pain but decreasing her overall health. She developed Chronic Fatigue Syndrome (CFS), Fibromalgia, diabetes, and intestinal problems. Her medications included four different anti-depressant drugs, high blood pressure medication, and several other drugs to offset the side effects of her required drug therapy and amounted to two hundred dollars a month.

After reflecting on Becky's illnesses, my mind returned to the present, and I wondered where the doctor was. It seemed like I had been waiting a long time. I reflected on the doctor's seminar talks as he had explained the Yin-Yang concept as the most basic concept of Chinese medicine. I could visually see him waving his hands in the air as he explained, "All things in the Universe are either Yin or Yang—nothing is ever all Yin or all Yang, but an ever-changing balance between the two. Chinese medicine treats illness by rebalancing Yin and Yang through acupuncture/acupressure, herbs, and Qigong, the oldest and most commonly used energy exercise."

"Chinese medicine believes the body has an energy force running through it called Qi, sometimes called life force or vital force. Qi or vital force is both matter (blood) and energy (Qi) and runs through channels, called meridians. If the flow of Qi along the meridians is insufficient, then Yin and Yang become unbalanced, resulting in illness. Blood transports Qi and nourishment."

The OMD had summarized Qigong as an Oriental therapy that combines gentle exercises with breathing techniques, meditation, and visualization to improve circulation of Qi in the body. What stood out most prominently in my memory was this statement that Qigong is especially beneficial for elderly people who wish to maintain flexibility and fitness!

I had done my own research on Qigong prior to this visit and learned that the history of Chinese Qigong is believed to date back to B.C. when Buddhism meditation methods were introduced from India and was practiced as a religion. Several hundred years later it was discovered that Qigong could be used for military purposes. Around 50 A.D. the Chinese emperor became a Buddhist and many meditation and Qigong practices that had been practiced in India for thousands of years were absorbed into Chinese culture and the training practices were recorded in Buddhist Bibles but kept secret and never taught to laymen. Shortly thereafter Tibetan Buddhist practices were also absorbed in China.

Further research into Chinese medicine revealed that the Chinese organized the world into five elements: Wood, Fire, Earth, Metal, and Water. They organized the body into corresponding systems with the five elements known as organ networks having different functions, but dependent upon each other to function properly. I learned that solid organs are Zang and hollow organs are Fu. The Zang-Fu organs are associated with specific body tissues and emotions.

If my memory served me correctly, the wood element is associated with the Zang organ, liver and the Fu organ, gallbladder. This was all so confusing to me because I did not consider my gallbladder to be hollow. "Isn't it the organ that produces bile?" I pondered. The specific body tissues associated with the liver are the eyes and tendons. I recalled the associated emotion as anger.

The fire element is associated with the Zang organ, heart and the Fu organ, small intestine. Again, I was puzzled—I definitely did not consider my small intestine hollow. The specific body tissues associated with the heart are the tongue and blood vessels. I recalled the associated emotion being joy.

The earth element is associated with the Zang organ, spleen and the Fu organ, stomach. Based on my appetite, I knew that my stomach could not possibly be hollow. The specific body tissues associated with the spleen are mouth and skin, and the associated emotion is pensiveness (absentmindedness).

The metal element is associated with the Zang organ, lungs and the Fu organ, large intestine. Its specific tissues are nose and skin and the associated emotion is grief.

The water element is associated with the Zang organ, kidney and the Fu organ, bladder. Its associated tissues are the ears and bones, and the associated emotion is fear.

What I think this all means is that if I have tendonitis, the Chinese might look for an imbalance in my liver and/or gallbladder rather than treating just the tendonitis. I grinned as I thought how mixed up American doctors might become trying to mix these philosophies with allopathic philosophies.

My reflections were interrupted when the door opened and a stream of light flooded the room as my doctor entered. To my relief, I clearly saw that the weird object was not a snake or an extra-terrestrial but an electrical device of some kind. I asked, "What is that crane-like device that has been staring at me?" He told me it was a device developed and known in China as the "Miracle Lamp."

The first thing the doctor did was to ask me for a health history. I told him about having had breast cancer, and that I was on a journey through alternative therapies to find detoxification and healing. He noted my concerns about the cancer returning in his chart notes. After the initial consultation, the doctor told me that he was going to use three therapies to increase my Qi, or vital energy. He explained that he would use acupressure to break up energy blockages in my meridians, Chinese visceral and lymphatic massage to break up congested lymph nodes and move lymph through my body to my liver and kidneys, and the far infrared mineral lamp to build up my Qi!

The energy guru explained that acupuncture is a popular form of therapy in TCM involving the use of sharp, thin needles that are inserted in the body at very specific points to adjust and/or alter the flow of energy and is used to treat many illnesses. Acupressure is a form of touch therapy that uses the principles of acupuncture and is a safe and effective way to reduce stress-related disorders such as headaches, ulcers, cramps, and insomnia by stimulating my own curative capabilities. Finger pressure is used instead of the insertion of needles to stimulate the acupuncture points. He emphasized that by using the power and sensitivity of the human hand, acupressure can be effective in the relief of tension-related ailments, self-treatment, and preventive health care.

The doctor continued his discourse, "Unmanaged stress and chronic tension are health hazards. It is believed that tension concentrates around acupressure points interfering with circulation and causing stagnation of the body flows in the nerves, blood vessels, and lymphatic ducts. Acupressure utilizes a system of points and meridians. The selected points used have a high electrical conductivity on the skin surface. Meridians are the pathways along which the body energy flows from point to point. Acupressure releases muscular tension and thus enables the blood to flow freely. This allows toxins to be released and eliminated. Acupressure also balances the emotions by releasing the emotions associated with tension usually caused by repressed feelings."

He grinned, "You will especially be interested in lymphatic drainage massage as it is used to increase the natural flow of lymph by elevating lymphatic circulation through the body's filtering systems, detoxifying the body and improving the immune system functions. Lymphatic massage is helpful to people suffering from lack of energy, a sluggish immune system, emotional stress, depression, and sports related injuries. It is very helpful to people who have had their auxiliary lymph nodes removed."

I did not know why he thought I would be interested in that because I still had my lymph nodes!

The energy guru continued, "There are three fluid circulatory systems of the body—the lymphatic system, blood circulation, and the cerebral-spinal fluid circulation. The lymphatic system consists of a system of ducts and vessels, lymph nodes, and lymph fluid. The functions of the lymphatic system are drainage and removal of fluid and waste products from the tissues. Networks of the lymphatic system are found in the neck, armpits, groin, pelvic area, along the windpipe, behind the abdominal cavity, and other places. When the body becomes congested, the lymph fluid becomes cloudy and thick."

He asked, "Have you ever had swollen glands in your neck that appear puffy?" I replied that I have had that condition several times throughout my life. The doctor explained, "These swollen glands are lymph nodes that have become congested from the build up of toxic waste and lack of blood circulation and lymph fluid and often are present with colds, allergies, and hay fever."

The body worker brought the far infrared mineral lamp over by the treatment table. With a close-up view, the device no longer frightened me. He told me the device was a far infrared mineral lamp and was called the "Miracle Lamp" in China. I looked for a light bulb in the device and could not find one? I asked, "Why is it called a lamp when it does not have a light bulb? He laughed and responded, "That is why it is called a miracle lamp." We both laughed!

He continued his discourse on lymphatic massage explaining that it is an excellent addition to every massage practice as it is gentle, and the rhythmic moves enables the therapist to massage swollen areas in the viscera that are difficult to do with other massage techniques such as Deep Tissue and Swedish massage.

With the explanations about his treatment modalities out of the way, he asked me to lie on my back. I was surprised since every body worker I had been to previously (mostly massage therapists and chiropractors) asked me to lay on my stomach. The doctor pulled up a stool, sat at the head of the table, and gently placed his hands under my head, feeling different areas at the base of my skull. I knew when he had found the specific spot he was looking for because I felt the pressure from his fingers push into my tissue. By looking upward as far as I could with my eyes, I could see his face. It appeared he was listening to my body flows as a traditional medical doctor would listen through a stethoscope. I asked, "What are you listening for." He responded that he was not listening—he was interpreting the energy with his other senses as it moved through my meridians." The healer explained that this technique was his most effective means of making a diagnosis. I was astounded! You can actually feel my energy?" I inquired. He grinned, "I pull your energy through my body." I thought he was joking with me again.

At the conclusion of the exploration of my energy field, I asked him what he had found. He told me that the energy flow in my body was stagnant, there were many blockages, and my liver was very congested. "You have a very high level of toxicity!" he added. At this time he turned the far infrared mineral lamp on. After allowing five minutes for the lamp to warm up, the body worker placed the head of the lamp about ten inches away from the vicinity of my liver. The warmth from the lamp felt good, and I could feel the energy from the lamp moving through my body. After a few minutes, I felt more relaxed.

The energy guru explained that the first technique he was going to use was acupressure to break up some of the blockages in my body. His hands were very soft, and I thought, "I am going to enjoy this as massage came to my mind." As his soft fingers found the first blockage in my neck and shoulder area, I realized I had misjudged those velvety, smooth hands when I winced from the pain inflicted on me. For several minutes, he applied pressure and massaged the swollen lymph nodes in an effort to break them up. I had not been aware of so many blocked and hot spots in my body. He continued the acupressure as he followed the meridians to my chest area. This time I screamed as he applied pressure to the blockages. The OMD explained that it was very important that I perform lymphatic massage in these areas often to keep the body flows moving, as routine lymphatic massage would help prevent breast cancer from occurring.

Other tender areas in my body were the meridians running up the inside of my thigh. It was excruciating as he broke up the blockages and moved the fluid. The energy guru pushed the far infrared mineral lamp to my right side while he worked on my left side. I told him the left side of my abdomen was very tender, and I was afraid I had developed a hernia or a cyst of some kind. After having had a cancerous tumor before, the fear of it returning was always there. The doctor located the lump that was causing the discomfort. He identified it as a congested lymph node. I was surprised and asked, "How do you know it is only a lymph node?" He told me it was his business to know such things. After several minutes of visceral massage, the pain was gone and so was the lump. I was impressed!

He then centered the far infrared mineral lamp on my liver and proceeded to work on my feet. The lamp was so soothing and comforting that I almost went to sleep. I asked him what made the lamp work. He told me the following story.

There was a one hundred-year-old ceramic factory in rural China in which there had been no reported arthritic complaints and other work-related pains from employees working in a poor environment where they had to work in black clay. In the early 1970s, the Chinese government sent a scientific team to investigate the factory. The scientists found that the black clay at the factory contained special healing elements. The far infrared mineral lamp was developed to mimic the properties of the clay.

The doctor told me the lamp is different from other infrared devices because the key component of the lamp is its heat-treated black plate that contains thirty-three different essential mineral elements used by the human body. The ceramic plate emits special spectrum-electromagnetic waves in the infrared range of 2 to 25 microns, compatible with bio-spectrum waves released by the human body, allowing the body to absorb the energy and use it to promote metabolism, regulate physiological deficiencies, diminish inflammation, and ease pain. I asked, "Can you explain why the special spectrum-electromagnetic waves produced by the far infrared mineral lamp work?"

He replied, "All life—plant, animal, and human—exists in a magnetic field and respond to the magnetic field of the Earth. Most animals exhibit a "homing instinct." Migratory birds fly south in the winter and salmon are magnetically guided back to their birthplace. Research shows animals respond to and are influenced by changes in the Earth's magnetic fields."

The lamp had relaxed me to the point that it was hard for me to stay awake. I wanted to let go and drift away on the big, fluffy cloud that I imagined I was on. My dream was interrupted as the energy guru continued, "The human body itself is electromagnetic (magnetism developed by electricity). Each body cell has a positive and negative field in the DNA. The human body cells are paramagnetic (capable of aligning with a magnetic field, but not becoming magnetized) and assume the polarity (the quality or condition of having two poles) of the magnetic field in which they exist. Tissue groups such as the central nervous system (the part of the nervous system consisting of the brain and spinal cord) and peripheral (outside the brain and spinal cord) tissues take magnetic polarities opposite to each other. All physical and mental energy in the human body and body functions are controlled by chemical electromagnetic impulses to and through the brain and central nervous system."

From this description of a human being, I saw myself in a completely different light—more like a robot than fleshy. He continued, "When considering that man is an electromagnetic creature with every cell in the living system an electrical battery and the function of the organs, glands, etc., electrochemical in operation, it becomes obvious that disorders and diseases are the result of electrochemical breakdowns that can be positively affected with appropriate application of electromagnetic therapies such as the far infrared mineral lamp."

I asked, "Are you saying that a device such as the far infrared mineral lamp can be used to treat cancer and other degenerative diseases with the energy it emits?" He replied, "Energy is essential to everyone with no respect of persons—the poor as well as the rich, the old as well as the young, and the sedentary as well as the athletic. Where does energy come from and where does it go? In order to answer these questions, it must first be understood that physical and mental energy are in reality, magnetic energy!"

He inquired, "Can you tell me some ways in which your body produces energy?" I told him by eating food. He continued, "Yes, magnetic energy is produced in several ways. One of the major sources of physical and mental energy is, of course, the biochemical processing of food and water by the body into energy. As food is eaten, salivation begins the chemical breakdown of the food, digestive processes continue, nutrients are absorbed into the blood, cells, nerves, etc., and ultimately produces electromagnetic energy—the energy of life."

"Life involves a multitude of physical and mental responses, all governed by electromagnetic energy—sight, hearing, movement, sensation, and metabolic processes, cell health, emotions, and thought. Therefore, from the biochemical standpoint, physical and mental functions are dependent on efficient digestion, absorption, and chemical process of foods and nutrients."

He asked, "Are you aware of other ways human energy is obtained?" I told him no. He continued, "A degree of human energy is inhaled via oxygen, derived through bone stress, electromagnetic energy produced from flexion and stress during exercise, and from red spectrum light in sunrises and sunsets."

He then explained that the functions of the far infrared electromagnetic mineral lamp are regulating metabolism, diminishing inflammation, easing pain, and that the lamp is extraordinarily effective in treating soft tissue injuries, arthritis, stomachaches, and skin conditions.

I asked him how the lamp differed from other electromagnetic and infrared devices. He replied, "As I mentioned earlier, the lamp features a black plate coated with a proprietary mineral formation consisting of thirty-three elements essential to the human body. When activated by a built-in electric heating element, this mineral plate emits a special band of electromagnetic wave ranging from 2 to 25 microns in wavelength that produces irradiation. This unique wavelength and output of energy makes the far infrared mineral lamp different from other far infrared energy devices and microwave therapeutic devices in that its electromagnetic waves coincide with the wavelengths and intensity of the electromagnetic waves of the human body and are consequently absorbed by the body. This absorbed electromagnetic energy has been found to yield therapeutic effects on the human body by helping to generate various beneficial biochemical stimuli that the body lacks due to illness, accident, or injury and by accelerating the decomposition of dead cells while enhancing body immunity."

He continued, "The lamp has shown breakthrough beneficial results in clinical and healthcare practice, agricultural production, and veterinarian care. The far infrared mineral lamp has been used on millions of patients in China and has been proven in a wide range of applications with high and immediate therapeutic results and with patients experiencing no pain." I thought, "Wow!" That piece of information increased my interest in the lamp—I do not like pain.

He then told me that the far infrared mineral lamp could be used in place of moxabustion. Moxabustion is the process in which moxa, a dried herb, is burned directly on the skin or just above the skin and over specific acupuncture points. When lit, moxa burns slowly, providing a penetrating heat that enters the channels (meridians) to increase Qi and blood flow.

The energy guru continued, "Life's energy is not a single energy but is a balance of two distinctly separate energies—negative magnetic energy and positive magnetic energy. Humans are electromagnetic organisms plugged into the magnetic fields of the earth, sun, and moon. Therefore, it is very important to be aware of the sources of biological magnetic energy such as the far infrared mineral lamp since there is a capability to alter these factors for the better."

When the treatment ended, the doctor sold me some Chinese herbs to cleanse my body and help build up my Chi. He reiterated that that Traditional Chinese Medicine (TCM) is a five thousand-year-old holistic approach to healing that helps the body's vital energy flow and is based on the theory that the body is electrical and chemical. These two forms of energy can be helped through acupressure (electrical energy field) and herbal teas or compounds (chemical energy field). Acupressure and herbs work together to promote and stimulate the natural healing mechanisms of the human body to restore and maintain good health.

My session with him was over. When it was time for me to leave, he gave me a hug. I smiled as I walked into the waiting room, pass the next client, and out into the gray Seattle drizzle.

I was determined to learn more about energy therapy. I found two good books describing the human energy field and its bio-magnetic nature: *Vibrational Medicine* by Richard Gerber, M.D., and *The Body Electric: Electromagnetism and the Foundation of Life* by Gary Selden et al today.

In Vibrational Medicine, Dr. Gerber states that conventional medical wisdom is being misguided by the concept that repairing or eliminating a body part with drugs and surgery can cure illnesses. He talks about how vibrational medicine attempts to treat people with pure energy instead of the conventional therapies of drugs and surgery. He discusses how this evolving field of science will bring doctors to a new level of understanding as it attempts to heal illness and transform human consciousness by working with the patterns that guide the physical expression of life since consciousness itself is a form of energy that is related to the physical body's cellular expression.

In the book, *The Body Electric: Electromagnetism and the Foundation of Life,* Robert O. Becker, M.D. a pioneer in the field of bioelectric science portrays the role electricity plays in healing. The book presents case studies and experiments on how bioelectricity and regeneration offer new approaches to healing cancer and other diseases.

2

FIR Mineral Treatments

I continued to see the oriental medical doctor. He used the far infrared mineral lamp in each session. While instructing me again on the benefits of the lamp, he asked me to work on developing body awareness. At the beginning of each appointment, he would ask me what part of my body felt the most depleted. On this particular day, the osteoarthritis in my right knee was bothering me. I pointed to my right knee. He agreed and placed the lamp over my knee and responded, "Kara, you are developing body awareness!" I thought it didn't take much awareness to know that my knee hurt.

The heat from the lamp felt good. I found the tension leaving my body, and soon I was relaxed and at ease. The heat had a comforting effect on my whole body. While my knee was receiving deep heating from the far infrared mineral lamp, the doctor was performing lymphatic massage on other parts of my body.

In every session with the doctor, in addition to the far infrared mineral lamp therapy, the doctor used Chinese visceral & lymphatic therapy. "Kara," he said, "The lymphatic system is the foundation of your immune system. Since your body has already proven it can develop cancer, you need to pay special attention to what I am going to tell you." He explained the following concepts to me.

"Not only is lymphatic drainage a key to disease prevention and rejuvenation, but also the means of contributing to the natural healing processes of the mind and body. It aids in the recovery of illness, weight loss, and overall body appearance. The proper functioning of the lymphatic system is critical to your body's ability to detoxify and regenerate tissues, filter out toxins, and maintain a healthy immune system."

The doctor talked about toxicity, "Western medicine has few tools to address toxicity since one can't operate or give a pill to detoxify the body." He suggested that pesticides are the primary toxins found in food, air, and water. He continued, "Pesticides cannot be seen or smelled—they attack the central nervous system and contribute to many neurological and mental health problems." As he talked, I thought about the effect car exhaust had on my nervous system. It was a cheap drunk for me. All I had to do was drive through heavy traffic and within a few minutes I would either be derisively happy or irritated and angry.

I knew exactly what he was talking about as I have suffered from environmental sensitivities most of my life. I also knew the side effects of detoxification. My body was very toxic and previous attempts at detoxifying had made me more ill as the toxins were being released from my tissues into my blood stream. I asked, "How are you going to protect me from the side effects of the released toxins when you are performing lymphatic massage on my body for an hour and a half?" As he adjusted the far infrared mineral lamp he said, "The concept of energizing the body while detoxifying is a vital and important principle in preventing poisoning the body; hence, the reason for using far infrared mineral therapy in conjunction with the lymphatic massage."

I was still curious as to how the far infrared mineral lamp emitted energy that the human body could absorb and use. I asked the doctor for more information on this process. He replied, "When the lamp was first introduced here, it was mistakenly referred to as far infrared therapy. It is much better than far infrared therapy. Bio-spectrum represents the broad energy spectrum that living organisms emit, sometimes referred to as an "aura," This lamp uses a blend of minerals (exactly in the spectrum of the minerals already present in the body) to create an infrared electromagnetic emission that is absorbed by the body. This emission of absorbable energy penetrates about into the body and causes what has been referred to as a resonance of the body's minerals, releasing the minerals from an oxidized condition, and making them available for use by the body. The far infrared mineral lamp reinforces the human body energy, improving health and the body's own self-healing functions."

After using the far infrared mineral lamp on my knee for about thirty minutes, I was amazed at the results. The stiffness and pain was gone from both knees. I felt heat throughout my body. I felt energized! The doctor explained, "The lamp relieves muscular aches and pains caused by arthritis and soft tissue injuries and is also effective in treating bone fractures."

While he worked on the rest of my body, I reflected on the information and knowledge I had learned about osteoarthritis, its cause, and therapies.

For those of us who suffer from arthritis, the daily tasks of climbing stairs, writing a letter, or standing at the sink washing dishes by hand can be a painful task. Osteoarthritis is by far the most common form of arthritis and is associated with the degeneration from the wear and tear of joints, as we get older. Risk factors for this ailment are age, nutritional deficiencies, tobacco and alcohol use, and obesity.

Western conventional therapies include the use of anti-inflammatory drugs to alleviate the pain. Some professionals believe these drugs may actually accelerate the degeneration of articular surfaces, necessitating replacement surgery. These drugs also can have serious side effects such as gastritis, ulcers, and kidney problems.

As a complimentary therapy, glucosamine is often prescribed. I reflected on how my alternative cancer doctor prescribed it for my painful knees. The healing benefits of glucosamine can take several weeks before improvement is noticed. The body uses glucosamine to manufacture and repair damaged connective tissue, resulting in greater joint integrity. I grinned as I recalled my allopathic medical doctor cautioning me about using it, "Glucosamine has not been evaluated by the FDA for safety, effectiveness and purity. All potential risks and/or advantages of glucosamine are not known, there are no regulated manufacturing standards in place for it, and there have been instances where herbal and health supplements have been sold containing toxic metals or other drugs." (These cautions serve medical doctors and the related pharmaceutical industry very well because they deter many people from trying any alternative healing technique.)

The energy guru interrupted my reflections as he proceeded to tell me how he viewed the causes of osteoarthritis. He focused his attention on my right foot and commenced with a teaching discourse. "Kara, as I have discussed with you before, the condition of the internal organs is closely related to osteoarthritis. As we discussed during your first visit, the five Yin organs, the heart, liver, lungs, kidneys, and spleen are most important for your health and long life and are interrelated. Whenever any of these organs is not functioning properly, illness and even death can occur."

He lapsed into another silence as he continued with the acupressure and lymphatic massage. I wondered which of my internal organs he was concerned with. I continued with my reflections of what I already knew. I knew that diet had a great deal to do with osteoarthritis in my knees. My naturopathic doctor had constantly urged me to rotate my foods as blood allergy tests revealed I have food allergies. She had talked to me about removing foods from my diet that cause inflammation such as dairy products, wheat, and the nightshade family (potatoes, peppers, eggplant, and tomatoes. I found it very difficult to follow her instructions because I loved wheat, dairy, and potatoes. In his efforts to prevent my body from developing another cancer tumor, my alternative medical doctor had urged me to eat very little animal protein other than fish and to eat a diet consisting of seventy percent vegetables.

Fasting speeds up the elimination and cleansing of the lungs, kidneys, liver, and even the skin. Fasting gives the digestive system a rest and relaxes the nervous system. Even my church teachings encourage me to fast once a month. I felt ashamed as I realized I have gained a lot of knowledge over the years—I just haven't had the will power and self-discipline to apply what I have learned.

My mentor stopped the bodywork and stared at me. I felt like I had no secrets from him, and from the look on his face, I sensed that I was in for a chastisement. "Kara," he said, "Weak joints can be the result of heredity or from the lack of exercise. Your weak knees can be strengthened by exercise. Qigong is a perfect exercise for you. When you exercise, Qi or energy is created at the joint from the movement of the muscles, tendons, and ligaments and will nourish the joint and rebuild it."

Remembering his discourse from our first encounter, I silently thought, "I can continue being lazy and indulge in foods that I love if I purchase a far infrared mineral lamp for my use at home. Didn't the OMD explain that the far infrared mineral lamp emits energy the body can absorb and use just like energy acquired from eating and exercising? Maybe I could have the best of both worlds—calories and nutrition.

My session with him was over. When it was time for me to leave, he gave me a hug. I smiled as I walked into the waiting room, pass the next client, and out into the beautiful Seattle sunshine.

3

Purchasing the FIR Mineral Lamp

I looked around the classroom. There were about twelve other people, mostly chiropractors. My co-worker and I were the only lay people in the class. The OMD had encouraged me to take his Chinese Visceral & Lymphatic Therapy class so I could learn to do lymphatic massage on others and myself. I felt good being there with chiropractors and other professional therapists—it did wonders for my self-esteem.

My mentor was expounding again, "Like a river, body energy must flow freely to avoid destruction and pain. Pain is caused by blocked energy!" He looked directly at me and said, "The four major components that impede the flow of the lymphatic system are: energy blockages or lack of energy, stress, in-active life style, and toxicity." I felt like I must stand out as I had all of them!

Concentrating on what he was saying was difficult for me as I was preoccupied with buying a far infrared mineral lamp. My appointments with the OMD were farther and farther apart. I was not making the necessary changes in my life style to obtain better health. Upon completion of this seminar, I would have all the training needed to do lymphatic massage on myself, but not have a means of getting energized and detoxifying the toxins when they were released as was provided in his treatment sessions. I felt I needed the far infrared mineral lamp in my home. The lamp was very expensive, and I had spent my savings on the registration for the class. I had to find a way to get my health care insurance to reimburse me.

Upon realizing that my thoughts were not on what was being said in the classroom, I forced myself to pay attention. The doctor was really absorbed in what he was sharing with the class. He continued, "Lymph fluid moves in one direction through a system of paired one-way valves in the lymphatic vessels. The lymphatic system has no central pump equivalent to the heart; therefore, movement is primarily accomplished by muscle contraction."

My mind turned back to the preoccupation of buying a lamp—my naturopathic doctor would need to write out a prescription for me to use the lamp for treatment of the osteoarthritis in my knees. The FDA accepted and approved the far infrared mineral lamp for use in the United States in 1988. The lamps are classified as an infrared lamp under Federal Regulations (21 CFR 890.5500) and have been assigned a CPT code, 97026, enabling doctors to bill insurance providers.

I again focused my attention on the doctor as he pointed to a chart showing the lymph system in a woman and said, "It is estimated that in a twenty-four hour period, forty-two pints of serum-like fluid passes from the bloodstream to body tissues carrying oxygen and nutrients and thirty-six pints return to the bloodstream carrying carbon dioxide and certain waste products. The remaining six pints pass from the tissues to the lymphatic capillaries carrying the majority of waste products and toxins."

I was getting hungry and wondered how long it was going to be before we ate lunch. Other students begin to stir. My attention immediately focused on the instructor as he was winding up his presentation and stated, "Energy moves the lymphatics; therefore, we are going to work with energy first—develop your intuition and awareness—approach your work with love and an open mind."

He gave instructions to choose a partner. We were going to learn by working on each other. My coworker and I formed a team and since there were an uneven number of people, we ended up with a young colon therapist on our team, too. The three of us would take turns working on each other.

The energy guru continued with, "Remember the concept of energizing the body while detoxifying it and always keep in mind to open the "gates." He described gates as blockages in front of and in the direction of where a body worker is working. He instructed us to open the gates to give the toxins and energy a place to move through. We were encouraged to balance our own energy first. My coworker and I both raised our eyebrows. I used the only tools I had in this category—affirmations and meditation. Hey, I presented a good of image of knowing what I was doing!

We were now ready to start lymphatic drainage. The OMD instructed us to first warm our hands and apply lotion or oil, start with a very light and gentle touch, moving very slowly, and work with the patient's knees up to relax the abdominal muscles. We were warned not to cross the abdominal mid-line with any pressure because of the major nerves and blood vessels that lay near the surface.

My coworker and I teased the male colon therapist and he loved it—it wasn't everyday he had two women working on his body. We were instructed to start on the patient's right side and make sure his/her knees were in an upright position. The first step was to start in the lower right corner of the abdomen (ascending colon) and follow the ascending colon slowly up to and under the right rib cage. We were to proceed along the transverse colon (the part of the colon that goes across the abdomen from right to left and is located between the ascending colon and the descending colon) until reaching the mid-line of the body, where we were to lighten the pressure to just skin touch and proceed to the spleenic flexure, continuing down the descending colon to the sigmoid colon.

When it was the colon's therapist's turn to work on my body, I gave him a bad time. There were instances when the student being worked on (me) was supposed to confirm that the procedure was done correctly. The colon therapist was doing a perfect job, and I could not stand it. So, on one particular procedure I continued to tell him he wasn't doing it right. He was frustrated! After the third try he caught on to my untruthfulness and promised to get even with me.

We spent the first day working on the upper body—the second day was scheduled for work on the lower part of the body. It was fairly easy to remain modest and covered during the bodywork training on the upper part of the body because we were allowed to keep our loose fitting tops on.

Working on the lower part of the body was a different story. The following day as I listened to the instructor's directions on how we were supposed to do the lymphatic massage on the lower body I realized it was going to be an invasive and humiliating procedure. Modesty would have to go out the window when my lower body clothing was removed. I decided I did not want some strange man pushing my lymph up my inner thigh and through the gates (lymph opening) in my groin. I feigned illness and left right before the exercise began.

My coworker ended up with a chiropractor from Eastern Washington as her partner. The following day I asked her how it went. She told me it was very invasive, she felt violated, and wished she had left when I did. For this reason, husband and wife teams are encouraged.

I gained a lot of knowledge and skills from attending the seminar and was grateful for the opportunity to pretend for one and a half days that I was a health professional. Neither my coworker nor I received the visceral therapy training, which was the last item of training in the seminar. Visceral therapy, known also as visceral manipulation, is the removal of restrictions in the soft tissue of the internal organs. When organs bind to each other or to the surrounding fascia, the organ cannot function properly. I had already learned a lot about this type of therapy because the OMD used it on me during each session. He taught that toxins have a big effect on the viscera. Many chronic conditions in other areas of the body refer to the viscera.

After attending the seminar, I made an appointment with my naturopathic doctor. She wrote a prescription for the far infrared mineral lamp. I submitted it to my insurance company and was reimbursed eighty percent of my cost. It was difficult finding a vendor to purchase the far infrared mineral lamp from. My coworker and I ended up purchasing the lamps through the OMD. The only drawback with this was that we had to wait until he came back into the area to get our lamps.

After several weeks of waiting, I received a phone call from the energy guru notifying me that he had my lamp. I made the appointment to see him—this session with the OMD marked a turning point in my journey to find healing, since I would be taking more control of my health care than ever before. Having access to the far infrared mineral therapeutic lamp in my own home was exciting and empowered me with confidence of a possible safe and healthy, pain-free future.

My mentor showed me how to assemble the lamp. It was very easy. He then spoke in his usual soft manner about using it, "You must be careful and cover your eyes with a cotton cloth or something similar when using the lamp for facial treatments. The part of your body being treated must be bare. Don't touch the lamp head during operation as it is very hot—keep children away from the lamp when it is in use."

My attention span was short, and I visualized myself lying under it with patches over my eyes. "I could use it to treat the white heads on my face," I thought. After all, the lamp was supposed to be very effective in treating skin conditions. He continued, "Protect the lamp against percussions and dampness. I wondered how I could protect the lamp against dampness—the Cascade foothills can almost qualify as a rain forest. It is difficult to keep the mold off the sidewalks and the house.

My mentor continued, "Keep the plate intact and do not clean with any type of liquid." I should have taken this warning to heart! Months later I let a friend take my magic lamp home with him to try out. He kept it for several weeks. When he returned the lamp the black plate was no longer intact as I could see the light from the interior. When I tried using the lamp, it had adverse effects. When I applied it to my weak foot, the ankle and foot swelled. Every time I used it, I developed complications. I suspect my friend removed the plate to see how it was put together and was not able to put it back together properly. The lamp squeaked when I adjusted the lamp head for different angles. I suspect my friend may have carried the lamp in his car over a period of time and the lamp was exposed to moisture. I decided to replace the lamp rather than replace the black plate because I do not know how the lamp was handled when it was out of my control. That was a learning curve. I am still willing to share the miracle lamp with others; however, the lamp stays in my possession and under my control!

The energy guru continued with his instructions, "Make sure the voltage requirements of the lamp match those of the power outlet before inserting the plug." Many electrical outlets in the United States operate on 100-volt electric current while outlets in the rest of the world operate on 220 volts or 240 volts. If a converter is required, make sure the appropriate adapter plug is used. The TDP lamp has the third grounding pin and should be used with three-pin grounded adapter plugs." An adapter won't change the electrical voltage—a voltage converter may be required.

I understood his concerns in this area. While employed as a safety director, the electrical receptacle outlets in the building were checked routinely. The most effective protection against electrocution is by installing ground-fault circuit interrupters (GFCIs). Electrical outlets can wear out from the repeated use of plugging and unplugging appliances. If the electrical plug fits loosely into the outlet or slips out of the outlet, the outlet may overheat and cause a fire hazard.

Remembering another important warning, the energy guru turned to me and said, "The plate lasts about seven hundred hours and then loses some of its effectiveness. After fifteen hundred hours the mineral plate must be replaced." I asked, "Do I have to record every minute I use it?" He replied, "It will take you many years to use fifteen hundred hours—don't worry about logging each time you use it."

We discussed the many conditions the lamp is effective in treating. One of my major interests was the relief of muscular aches and pains caused by arthritis. I was visualizing how good it would feel to use the lamp after a hike. Again, the OMD interrupted my thoughts, "You can use the lamp to alleviate inflammation and edema from soft tissue injuries. Remember, the lamp can promote healing effects on internal organs, and you can balance your nervous system with the lamp! Oh, and one last thing—if you ever break a bone, you can use it to treat the bone fracture—but, I recommend that you see a qualified doctor first."

I thought, "All of this information was nice, but how would I know how many sessions and for how many weeks to treat a broken bone?" The doctor was right. I should use self-therapy with discretion and always get a doctor's opinion for such a serious condition as a broken bone.

After covering all the important issues regarding the lamp that he thought was important, he asked, "What area of your body do you think we should direct the lamp at tonight?" I pondered his question for a minute and replied, "I think we should direct the lamp at my liver because, according to what you have taught me about Traditional Chinese Medicine, the imbalances in my liver and other internal organs are probably most responsible for the arthritis in my knees. He laughed and said, "You are a very good pupil, and we will use the lamp on your liver tonight."

My session with him was over. When it was time for me to leave, he gave me a hug. I smiled as I walked into the waiting room carrying my far infrared mineral lamp, pass the next client, and out into the unique Seattle breezes.

4

FIR Mineral Energy

Since attending the energy guru's seminars, I spent considerable time researching and learning as much as I could about the far infrared mineral lamp. I learned that far infrared energy in used therapeutically in many different ways. Probably the most common usage is for pain relief and healing.

In China, the far infrared mineral lamp has been proven to be especially effective as a treatment for pain relief in various muscular-skeletal ailments and injuries. This non-invasive device is very effective in the treatment for chronic pain experienced in backaches, fibromyalgia, arthritis, and similar soft tissue problems because of their vasodilatation qualities—increased blood flow and local temperature. This action brings nutrients and oxygen to the soft tissue area while stimulating the removal of accumulated toxins.

It seems to me that the far infrared mineral device accomplishes some of the same actions as exercise. I recalled some of the procedures and techniques I had learned while employed as a safety director in a small manufacturing plant. One technique used in preventing carpel tunnel and other work-related injuries was to implement more mini breaks with fast moving exercises such as walking swiftly down the hall and back to the employee's desk. I remember one of the women ran up and down the outside steps to the building several times during her mini breaks. The Department of Labor & Industries' physical therapist suggested that these fast-action mini breaks would accomplish two things—increase the blood flow resulting in increased nutrition to these weakened body parts and remove the accumulated toxins. I believe the far infrared energy does a little more than exercise—supposedly it reduces levels of lactic acid, a by-product of muscle metabolism that causes pain and stiffness following exercise.

My understanding is that some of the early Chinese scientist involved in the development of the far infrared mineral energy device characterized its healing power as resonant absorption, meaning the tissues selectively absorb the rays. I think resonant absorption means that the far infrared mineral rays naturally generate heat by causing the body's molecules to rapidly vibrate against each other. These scientists believed that the human body tissues produce infrared energy that is associated with many different healing functions and that the far infrared mineral devices provide a boost to the body's production of it. It is believed that after the body's production of far infrared energy is maximized, the remaining energy passes away without any harmful side effects. I liked this idea—no damaging side effects!

The far infrared mineral lamp's healing effects are comparable to the healing powers of various kinds of the laying-on-of-hands techniques, some of which date back thousands of years. In the first chapter, I discussed somewhat the history of Qigong. I recall that an important principle of Traditional Chinese Medicine is that good blood circulation promotes good health. Supposedly the ancient Qigong healers had the ability to emit energy through their hands. Modern scientific researchers believe that this ancient form of energy medicine was based on the premise that the human body itself radiates infrared rays. The Bible contains many incidents in which Jesus Christ healed many different types of ailments through the technique of hand touching. There was even one instance in which a woman was healed just by touching his garments. After his death, his disciples continued healing by the laying on of hands.

5

Using the Lamp

I found that the far infrared mineral lamp is great for soft tissue injuries—sprains, strains, pulled tendons, stretched ligaments, and all the other painful traumatic things that will happen to us at various times in our lives, including the painful effects of arthritis.

I recommend that if a person desires to use the far infrared mineral lamp to treat a disease or an illness they consult an Oriental Medical Doctor (OMD) or a physician of their choice for diagnosis and identification of the problem before trying self-treatment with the lamp. The far infrared mineral lamp comes with instructions that list contraindications for its use. Some diseases to use caution with in self-therapy are adrenal suppression, Lupus erythemastosus, and multiple sclerosis.

Adrenal suppression probably indicates a condition in which the adrenal glands perform low adrenal output. At one time tuberculosis was classified as the number one cause of adrenal insufficiency. Today the number one cause is the use of steroids followed by fungal infections as the number two cause of adrenal insufficiency, which can be a life threatening chronic illness.

Lupus erythemastosus is a disorder of the immune system in which the body harms its own healthy cells and tissues causing inflammation and damage to various body tissues. Some of the most common symptoms are extreme fatigue, painful or swollen joints (arthritis), skin rashes, kidney problems, and unexplained fevers. There is no cure for lupus.

Multiple sclerosis is an inflammatory disease affecting the central nervous system. MS victims can experience partial or complete loss of any function that is controlled by, or passes through, the spinal cord and brain.

After I first obtained the lamp, I was eager to share information with others based on my own experiences and failed to take into account other people's lifestyles. For example, I do not use drugs of any kind so I do not think about the possible effects far infrared mineral therapy might have on someone that uses a huge amount of prescription or non-prescription drugs. If a person is using many prescription drugs, I think that they might want to consult with their physician or pharmacist to ensure that the far infrared mineral lamp will have only positive interaction with the drugs. Rarely do doctors prescribe only one drug—usually a person ends of with another drug to offset the side effects of the first drug, and on and on it goes until the medicine cabinet is full of prescription drugs.

Some people think it not advisable to treat an acute joint injury with the far infrared mineral lamp for the first forty-eight hours after an injury or until the swollen symptoms subside. I used the lamp early on and suffered no side effects. This type of heating may be contra-indicated in cases of enclosed infections. I did use the lamp on my gums after I had my two upper wisdom teeth removed, but I wondered about its effectiveness with tooth decay.

A friend of mine bought the far infrared mineral lamp about the same time as I did to treat a fungus infection. She had recently visited her homeland, the Philippines, and had been told by a family doctor to look for an infrared lamp to treat the fungus-infected bone in her foot. She was excited to purchase and try the lamp. Previously, doctors had used surgery to scrape the bone, hoping to destroy the fungus. As a result of the multiple surgeries the foot became deformed—antibiotics and other drugs were ineffective. She was very angry with the medical doctors for messing up her foot and was determined to heal the foot herself. She had fewer concerns about the potential risks of the infection being in an enclosed area in her bone than she did about the doctors performing additional surgeries.

Another area of treatment that might be questionable is an area that contains metal pins, rods, artificial joints, and other metal surgical implants that may reflect infrared rays.

As the far infrared mineral lamp increases blood flow, some women may not want to use the far infrared mineral therapy for low back pain during the menstrual period as it may increase the menstrual flow. I guess it is an individual thing—decrease pain and increase blood flow, or just suffer the pain of menstruation. Because of the increased blood flow from far infrared mineral therapy, hemophiliacs and those predisposed to hemorrhage may not want to use the far infrared mineral lamp.

When using the lamp, care should be given to ensure that nothing touches the lamp head during operation. The lamp should be protected against dampness and blows. The plate must be kept intact and not cleaned with any type of liquid.

When using the lamp for facial treatments, be sure and cover the eyes with a cotton patch or similar material. Small children should be kept away from the lamp when it is being used since the plate becomes very hot. My little granddaughter likes to turn the switch on an off, so I unplug it when it is not in use to prevent her from injuring herself.

Now that I have discussed the possible few negative concerns regarding the lamp I would like to talk about all the great positive things the lamp will do.

One of the first things I did after buying the far infrared mineral lamp was to discard all of the pain killers, antihistamines, aspirin, Tylenol, etc. from my medicine cabinet. It has always been a concern of mine when the grandchildren were around that one of them would get into a bottle of drugs and have to have his/her stomach pumped. My middle child did exactly that. She climbed upon the sink and took several of her father's allergy medicine tablets. We rushed her to the doctor's office—they pumped her stomach. I was asked to hold her while the doctor did this agonizing procedure. To this day, this daughter does not like to be physical in her relationships. She loves me—she just doesn't want me touching her. Parents need to be careful how they handle emergency situations and be sensitive to children's fears of being restrained.

As mentioned previously in this book, I first used my new far infrared mineral lamp on my knee. The ligaments in my right knee were always tender and the joint knocked and popped after walking a short distance. The heat from the far infrared mineral lamp felt good and enticed my whole body to relax. Within a few minutes, a good deal of the stress and tension was gone from my body. I have tried the lamp at different distances from my knee. Some people say the lamp should be six to eight inches from the body part being treated, others say a foot, and my mentor always placed it about a foot from the body part he was treating.

The lamp gets very hot when it is placed within six inches of the body part being treated. When determining the distance to place the lamp, I think of the advice the OMD always gave me, "If a therapy or modality is hurting you, stop using it!" So, I always move the lamp to the distance that is the most comfortable. For my first home treatment, I used the far infrared mineral lamp on my knee approximately twenty minutes twice a day for two weeks. I try to use moderation in all things and am reluctant sometimes to use the lamp for more than two weeks consecutively for fear that my body will get acclimated to the lamp and my body functions will slow down and/or shutdown because the need to function is replaced by the lamp. Opponents of daily vitamin therapy used to tell me that if I took vitamins every day for long periods of time my body would decrease its own activities of absorbing the vitamins from food eaten and rely on obtaining the nutrients from the vitamin supplements.

I use the far infrared mineral lamp to increase my energy level. On days when I am feeling angry or irritable, a few minutes under the lamp will transform me into a pleasant and happy person. The lamp is great for depression. I think depression and low energy go together. It is hard to be depressed when one is full of energy. The far infrared mineral lamp also works well when I have insomnia.

Many people have sleep disorders that prevents them from enjoying their life to its fullest. There are many causes of insomnia such as depression, stomach problems, caffeine, alcohol, worry, and drugs taken to stay awake. Other reasons for insomnia include taking daytime naps, exercising close to bedtime, watching TV late into the night, eating within an hour of bedtime, and irregular sleep schedules. Depression and worry are my major causes of insomnia.

I think all of us suffer with insomnia at some time in our lives from stress, jet lag and other problems. Insomnia sometimes increases with age and sometimes is a symptom of another medical disorder. Doctors prescribe sleeping pills for short-term insomnia—the pills usually quit working after several weeks of continuous use. Antidepressants are used both to induce sleep and treat depression.

Sleep apnea is another sleep disorder where breathing is interrupted. It is sometimes associated with fatty tissues or loss of muscle tone from aging. Loud snoring usually accompanies it. When trying to breathe, the windpipe collapses blocking airflow for ten seconds to a minute while the person tries to breathe. When the oxygen level drops in the person's blood, the brain awakes the person causing the upper airway muscles to tighten. The person then gasps and starts snoring again. Frequent awakenings leave people sleepy, irritable, with headaches, and depressed. Mild sleep apnea can be overcome by weight loss or sleeping on the side instead of the back. Sometimes surgery is used to treat the problem. I consider sleep apnea to be a serious situation. I worked with a lady who suffered with it, and I worried about her fearing what would happen if her body failed to wake up after the oxygen dropped.

I am sixty-four years old and rarely have a sleep problem. I attribute this to sleeping on a firm, good mattress. Replacing a mattress every six to ten years is a place to start to ensure a good night's sleep. I also sleep on a magnetic mattress pad. If you listen to "the opposition" they will tell you the same old rhetoric, "magnetic mattress pads have not been approved by the FDA to treat any medical condition, there is no evidence that they provide any benefits, and so on." I feel the pad helps me sleep deeply and soundly, waking up rested and energized. I try not to eat sugars for at least two hours before going to bed. I sleep with the window open a crack and make sure the temperature is around 60 degrees. I cannot stand to have a lot of clothing on so I only wear enough to be modest if I had to leave quickly.

Exiting the house in an emergency brings to my mind a recent experience. For the first time in my life I had a security system installed. It takes forty-five seconds for the alarm to sound when the front door is opened. The alarm sounds immediately when the back door in my daughter's room is opened. When using the security system for the first time, my daughter woke up coughing and felt she wanted to spit. Since her bed is very close to the outside door, she opened the door and spit out. The alarm went off immediately. I shot out of my bed! We both raced to the kitchen to turn off the alarm. The security company called within three minutes to see if we were all right. They laughed when I explained that my daughter opened the door to spit. It took me forty-minutes to get back to sleep. We really are careful not to trip that alarm.

I am so grateful that ninety-seven percent of the time I can fall asleep within twenty minutes and sleep soundly for five to six hours. The few nights that I cannot sleep are miserable. I have found that counting sheep does not work. If I have lain in bed for twenty minutes or more, my first offensive action is to take calcium and magnesium supplements, Vitamin B, and Vitamin C. If I have not fallen to sleep within twenty minutes after taking the food supplements, I move the far infrared mineral lamp over next to the bed, heat it up for five minutes, and then direct it on my stomach. Within twenty minutes, I usually feel relaxed and sleepy. The lamp shuts off automatically.

Recent research indicates that feelings of nausea are usually due to anxiety and depression rather than any serious medical problem. I have found that to be the case in dealing with my own stomach problems. The research also revealed that stomach ailments could be warning signs of emotional problems. Many people with insomnia seek professional help from their family doctor who places them on harmful medications after having run expensive, unnecessary medical tests because the real problem was anxiety and/or depression. As I mentioned earlier, when I start taking one medication, in a short time I found myself taking two or three others to combat the side effects caused by the first medication and it goes on and on. Starting on medication is one way to ensure that a medicine cabinet will fill up quickly.

My youngest daughter had some teenage friends who pretty much kept themselves in drugs such as Vicodin, which they combined with other substances and used for pleasure. They each took turns seeing a doctor for pain—each received a prescription for a goodly amount of the narcotic—enough to provide all with a good time.

Abdominal pain is often a symptom of indigestion or gas. Sometimes worms, bacteria, viruses, and tumors can cause stomach problems. Misalignment of the pelvic vertebrae can cause abdominal pain—this is why I see my network chiro-practor once a week—to keep those vertebrae in the right alignment!

An alternative to chemical drugs is naturopathic remedies such as oil massages containing mint, fennel or jojoba massage oil, gently massaged in circular motions on the stomach can soothe and calm an upset stomach caused by anxiety and stress. Herbal teas like chamomile tea are an effective stomach pain. I always have chamomile tea in stock. It is not only relaxing but allows me to snooze.

Certain foods and beverages are known to stimulate the stomach and produce excessive stomach acid while others weaken the esophageal sphincter, allowing food to back up into the esophagus. I have experienced this. I didn't even get a warning of a burp—it just erupted, and I had this foul tasting stomach residue in my mouth. This happens more at night because gravity may cause food and acid to back up more easily when one is lying down. Possible causes are late night snacks, nicotine, caffeine, milk, citrus fruits, peppermint, tomatoes, fried, fatty, and spicy foods, stressful situations, and obesity. These last three are the ones that really get to me. I recently read that sleeping on the left side helps because the right side worsens heartburn. I wonder if that is why I usually sleep on my left side.

Obesity is a major cause of stomach problems because it places excessive pres-sure in the area of the abdomen, pushing contents back up into the esophagus. Several weeks ago I was working with my trainer at a local gym. He wanted me to use a piece of equipment that required lying on my stomach and lifting weights up with my legs. When I first tried this, it forced stomach contents up through my esophagus. After several weeks of training and working out, I was able to per-form the exercise without the stomach backup. Studies show that exercise and weight reduction can reduce heartburn.

I find that the far infrared mineral lamp works wonderfully on stomach prob-lems. I usually place the lamp about a foot away from my stomach and turn it on for twenty minutes—other times I can use it longer. The heat from the lamp is so soothing, relaxing, and the absorbable energy directed at my stomach dissipates discomfort. Usually it is only a few minutes of far infrared mineral lamp therapy, and I am relaxed and ready to sleep soundly for the next six or seven hours.

The far infrared mineral lamp truly is a miracle!

6

Back Pain and FIR Mineral Lamp Therapy

I have suffered with back pain and have done considerable research on it. I have discovered that back pain is very difficult for doctors to diagnose because there are so many possible causes. Some indications of back problems are back pain with weakness or numbness in one or both legs, pain going down one leg below the knee, and back pain from an injury. Everyone's back pain is different—some have mild back pain and some have severe pain. Most back pain is acute (short-lived). My lower back bothers me the most, and I just love the heat from the far infrared mineral lamp. It is so relaxing and the time goes by too fast when I am using it.

Backache can be caused by pressure on back muscles or nerves. Illnesses, strains, sprain, and overuse can damage the spine. Emotional stress slows recovery and can even cause pain. I have been seeing a network chiropractor for two and one-half years for treatment of emotional problems that caused lower back and lower leg problems.

A ruptured or herniated disc can push into the spinal canal and puts pressure on the nerve roots, causing irritation. Back pain, muscle spasms, and sciatic pain can cause a disk to rupture. Sometimes surgery is used to treat this type of back problem—many times not helping the problem much at all.

Many back injuries are caused by a sudden twist or motion, resulting in muscle strain. Thin and weakened bones sometimes due to calcium loss cause Osetoporosis. The bones in the spinal column are fragile and break more easily, especially in older women. Osteoporosis, lifting heavy objects, or just moving the wrong way can cause compression fractures. Rheumatoid arthritis causes stiff, painful, and swollen joints in the neck. Some rheumatic disorders cause muscle pain and stiffness in the neck, shoulders, lower back, and hips.

Fibromyalgia can cause pain and stiffness in muscles and tendons, especially in the neck and upper back, and if often associated with sleep problems, lack of exercise, or an old injury.

Lack of exercise, poor posture, stress, and obesity contribute to back problems. Many people tighten back muscles when stressed. Obesity puts added pressure and strain on the back and stomach muscles, stretching and weakening them. Weak back and stomach muscles do not support the back properly, and poor posture shifts the body out of balance.

My workout program at the gym includes a warm-up period (thirty minutes of aerobic activity) three to four times a week, which will produce a slimmer waistline and healthier back when I use it on a regular basis.

Because I am older and overweight, I am familiar with back pain and weakened back and stomach muscles. For the treatment of a specific back pain from a strained or sprained muscle, I lay under the far infrared mineral lamp for twenty to forty minutes every day for ten to fourteen days in a row. As mentioned previously, I like to treat an area for two weeks, and then discontinue the far infrared mineral lamp for a week or so. The deep heat and absorbed energy not only relax and soothe my back, but strengthen the bones, muscles, and ligaments. The far infrared mineral lamp is the only modality I know of that will provide immediate relief from pain without harmful side effects.

A good percentage of the lower back pain I experience is referred from my kidneys. I believe I incurred some kidney damage from not drinking enough water for so many years. The OMD continually encouraged me to drink a gallon of water a day—at least! I find the far infrared mineral lamp very good for my congested kidney tissues. After applying the lamp to my kidneys, my urination frequencies increase for the next twenty-four hours. When my ankles are puffy and congested with fluid, I usually direct the head of the lamp to my lower back area, because I feel my swollen ankles are usually related to my kidney deficiencies.

I was ignorant for so many years of the importance of drinking enough, good quality water. The human body was created to function on water and minerals. I have found that when I used the far infrared mineral lamp on my body for more than twenty minutes, I must increase my water intake over the next twelve hours possibly because of the absorption of minerals from the lamp and the detoxification process that is occurring. I have read a lot over the last few years on how much the healing process depends on sufficient water intake. This is understandable as our bodies are over seventy percent water. Dr. F. Balmanghelidj wrote a good book on water intake entitled *Your Body's Many Cries for Water*. Dr. Balmanghelidj believes that chronic and persistently increasing dehydration is the root cause of almost all currently encountered major diseases of the human body. He is a medical doctor known for water cures. Prior to reading his book, I was always confused as to how much water to drink daily. The OMD encouraged me to drink at least a gallon on water a day. Dr. Balmanghelidj gives more individualized instructions as he suggests that I drink one-half of my body weight in ounces of water per day and add one-fourth teaspoon of salt to my diet for each quart of water I consume. Depending on how much I weigh, that might be a lot more than one gallon of water per day.

A few years ago my body was very toxic, and I was not drinking near enough water. My nervous system went crazy when I was exposed to chemicals. It was very difficult for me to drive in traffic. When my lymphatic system is congested and contaminated with chemicals, it affects my nervous system, and I suffer with many mental distortions such as anxiety, panic, slow thought process, and even exaggerated happiness. Today there is a lot of suspicion that many degenerative and neurological diseases and illnesses are caused by dehydration and toxicity. Based on my own experiences, I believe this to be very true. Some illnesses possibly related to dehydration are Chronic Fatigue Syndrome, anxiety, depression, Attention Deficit Disorder, and Alzheimer's disease.

Many people believe that water is the key to a longer life. I believe that drinking enough chemical-free water combined with adequate trace minerals can expand a human's life span. Just about every body function depends on adequate water intake—digestion and nutrient absorption, elimination, and even energy. I read that there is a link between insufficient water intake, weight gain, and malnutrition because the body absorbs carbohydrates rapidly and insufficient water intake can cause the body to absorb the calories without the nutrients.

I remember there was a period in my life when I got really sick. It was hard for me to eat any food and the weight started coming off very fast. I was not drinking enough water at the time, and I suffered terribly. I was very toxic and when the fat came off so did one heck of a bunch of toxins. I found that it was painful and even dangerous to detoxify my body without adequate water intake. If there is one thing that I have learned over the past several years, it is that detoxification is very important to being and staying healthy.

There are many books written on the importance of fasting, colon therapy, and juicing to eliminate toxicity including *Edgar Cayce's Guide to Colon Care: The First Step to Vibrant Health* by Sandra Duggan and *The Juiceman's Power of Juicing* by Jay Kordich.

Edgar Cayce is often referred to as the father of holistic medicine. He believed that all organs, glands, cells, and other tissues in the body are affected by the condition of the colon, and clearing the colon of toxins is the first step to increase physical energy and mental clarity. Colon hydrotherapy is a treatment employing detoxification equipment to inject warm water into the colon to release waste material and intestinal plaque resulting in blood and tissue detoxification and improved digestion.

People who have seen him on television know Jay Kordich as the "juiceman". In his book, he describes his program for staying healthy, looking young, and feeling great by using the natural healing power of fresh fruit and vegetable juices. He suggests fresh juice combinations that will help lower cholesterol, assist in weight loss, and reduce the risk of many serious diseases.

The quality of water is just as important as the amount. I buy a lot of bottled water and have a purifying unit in my home. Chlorine and other chemicals in water can also make a person ill. In addition, if the drinking water is saturated with chemicals, it has little ability to remove any toxins from the body—it just adds more pollution to the body cells and fluid.

Many times I find myself very tired. It is amazing how quickly I can become energized just from drinking water. The other night my friend and I were shopping. My knees hurt, my feet hurt, and my ankles were very swollen. I realized that my water intake had not been sufficient throughout the day. We stopped and bought a couple of bottles of water. A short time later, we stopped at a restaurant to get some food, and I was feeling more energetic and my body parts did not hurt so badly. I said, "Karolyn, my knees are not as sore." She laughed at me and said, "The water cannot work that fast." I said, "It takes less time for the soda pop you drink to run through you than this water that I have just consumed, so why do you think water cannot work that fast for me?"

I have been working out at a local gym with a trainer who insists that I bring plenty of water to drink. At the beginning of each session, he asks me if I have been drinking enough water. The man with a perfect body can always tell if I am dehydrated by my energy level. However, by the time the session is over I am no longer dehydrated. The trainer also tells me that I could lose weight just by drinking enough water. He always had a bottle of water with him while he worked with people and told me that the reason I could lose weight by drinking clean, pure water is because it increases nutrient absorption, weight loss, skin complexion, and helps detoxify the body. Wow, I am amazed and impressed that body builders and gym trainers know so much about good health—but that is their business to know!

The body builder challenged me to drink a specific amount of water each day for the next five days. I did—he was right. I dropped four pounds in those five days just by drinking enough water. The trainer explained that the weight loss was due to my liver converting fat into energy, and asked me if I ate as much during these five days as I usually did. I had to acknowledge that I had not because I did not have as much appetite. I have heard repeatedly that many times when one craves sugar or chocolate, they are really thirsty for water. The weight instructor said, "Kara, water speeds up your metabolism and a faster metabolism produces more energy which helps your body absorb nutrients better. He also encouraged me to take a multiple vitamin and mineral supplement daily to ensure my body was getting enough minerals.

I omitted telling him that my body was absorbing minerals from the far infrared mineral lamp in addition to the ones I was consuming through eating because I was using it more frequently when working out to ease the discomfort in my muscles.

7

Sprains & Strains

I have five daughters and they were very active in sports. My youngest daughter played just about every sport that was available. When she was very young, I started her in gymnastics. She had perfect form and was very flexible—she did very well in this sport. We lived in an incorporated town in Washington, and The Boys & Girls Club had a very good gymnastics program and very good volunteer instructors. I love to get out the photographs that show her walking and performing on the beam and doing her routines.

The Boys & Girls Club also had a very good soccer program for young children and very good volunteer instructors and coaches. My daughter learned to play soccer very well. She worked her way up to play on a very elite team, and I would dream of what she would accomplish in years to come.

Kelly's successful career in gymnastics and soccer ended when we moved to a rural community in the Cascade Foothills, miles from a gymnastics organization. The move helped me because I found nature very healing, but it sure put a crimp in my daughter's sports future. She was able to continue playing soccer, but on a much lower skill level then what she had been accustomed to.

Sprains, strains, and broken bones sometimes accompany young athletes, and my daughter certainly had her share. I did not have a far infrared mineral lamp during those years; consequently, she has injuries that have never healed properly. Ace bandages, Epsom salts, and ice bags were frequent accompaniments on our sports trips. Sometimes her injuries were called sprains and sometimes they were called strains. These are the most common sports injuries. I always marveled how the doctors could identify which one the injury was.

Orthopedic medicine describes a sprain as a stretch or tear of a ligament. A ligament can be described as the fibrous band of connective tissue that joins the end of one bone with another. The ligament helps stabilize and support joints. By the time my daughter graduated from high school, the ligaments in her ankles no longer supported or helped stabilize her ankle—they were stretched! She used the muscles in her limbs to support her in running. She was very limited in jumping skills.

A sprain is caused by a fall or other accidental trauma that knocks a joint out of position, overstretching and often rupturing the supporting ligaments. This occurred frequently when she along with two or three other players jumped in an effort to hit and direct the soccer ball with their heads. Often feet and legs would become tangled in the air, and she would land on the side of her foot upon touching the group. The weight on the turned-sideways foot would usually be that of two or three players. She rarely suffered from arm or hand strains. Even when sliding into bases while playing baseball, she only injured her ankles or knees.

A strain is described as a twist, pull, or tear of a muscle or tendon, the fibrous cords that attach muscles to the bones. She had fewer strains than sprains. I saw more strains while working as a safety coordinator in a small manufacturing plant. Chronic strains developed in the work environment from overuse, prolonged, and repetitive movement of muscles and tendons. In sports, a direct blow to the body, overstretching, or excessive muscle contraction can cause acute strains. Too often the school sports coaches lacked sufficient education and knowledge to properly teach the players how to stretch properly.

While my daughter was incurring these injuries continually, I was not knowledgeable enough to understand that my daughter was a risk for this type of injury because of her history of sprains. People in the general public are a risk if they are overweight and in poor physical condition; however, my daughter's weight was in proportion to her height and she was very healthy.

All sports and exercises bring a risk of sprains. Even walking! Many times while walking I have stumbled and stretched a muscle. The sports that my daughter loved to play the most were basketball and soccer in which much jumping was involved carrying a big risk for foot, leg, and ankle sprains. She tried just about every kind of ankle brace there was to try. Gymnastics carry a big risk for hand strains because of the extensive gripping, but she never developed these types of strains. She incurred maybe one strain while playing softball.

The symptoms of Kelly's sports injuries were bruising and inflammation, accompanied by pain. My daughter had a very high tolerance for pain. She would continue playing when peers with a similar injury would be out of the game and on the bench crying. With most of her ankle injuries she would feel a pop or a tear in the joint. Most of Kelly's sprains were severe, and she would feel an excruciating pain at the moment of injury as the ligament tore completely or separated from the bone, giving the joint very limited functioning. Sometimes it was only a moderate sprain, partially tearing the ligament and producing joint instability and swelling. Usually a ligament is stretched in a mild sprain, and there is no joint loosening.

After finishing the basketball season in her senior year, Kelly had surgery to correct her torn ligaments. Following the surgery she went to Russia for six weeks on an agricultural student exchange program. Upon returning to the United States, she was selected to play in the state high school girls' all-star team. While playing she sprained her ankles again, ripping out the stitching from the previous surgery and ending her basketball career.

Typical indications of strains are pain, muscle spasm, muscle weakness, swelling, inflammation, and sometimes cramping. The muscle and tendons are sometimes completely ruptured in severe strains. I incurred severe strains in my knee, while trying to walk with an injured foot. My knee hurt so bad I would cry all the way to work because it hurt so much to apply a small amount of foot pressure on the gas pedal.

Most common strains are in the back when the supporting muscles are twisted, pulled, or torn. My daughter incurred some back strain from jumping while playing basketball. Another common strain is the hamstring muscle strain in the back of the thigh, common in professional basketball and football players.

Rest, ice packs, braces, and elevation were the usual therapies for treating Kelly's sprains and strains from sports injuries. I can remember many trips to emergency rooms to ensure there were no broken bones. Usually, we saw an orthopedic surgeon—sometimes physical therapy was prescribed.

There are some exercises my daughter was encouraged to do to help prevent future injuries such as muscle strength and conditioning programs. The local high school had several weight lifting classes. I often wonder if the instructors had acquired enough knowledge to adequately teach those programs.

Another preventive technique was daily stretching exercises. I cannot recall ever seeing Kelly do these types of exercises. Her older sister, Renee, stretched on a daily basis and rarely incurred a sports injury. Other preventive measures are wearing properly fitting shoes and eating a well-balanced diet. My daughters always had high-priced, supportive shoes; however, the soda pop probably was not very nourishing. There was always a warm-up period before the sports activity and my daughters always arrived at activities early enough to get a proper warm up.

Today the far infrared mineral lamp is available to me to treat these kinds of injuries and can be used to increase the elasticity of collagen tissues in her sports injury.

8

Minerals & Absorption

As mentioned earlier, my trainer at the gym urges me to take a multivitamin everyday. The gym has their own brand of food supplements and fluids, and I have been using my own brand for many years because I know how important processing and raw materials are in the final product. Vitamins are very important, but they need the minerals for assimilation because minerals act as catalysts for many processes in the body. My multivitamin and mineral supplement is processed from alfalfa and other organic greens. Alfalfa is a very rich source of trace minerals. The alfalfa plant root grows deep into the soil where it extracts iron, calcium, potassium, important trace minerals and other elements from the subsoil areas.

Alfalfa can be taken in a tablet or capsule form. It can also be taken in a tea. Alfalfa helps the body to assimilate vital nutrients to build up immune function and is beneficial in helping the body break down carbon dioxide. It is purported to reduce cholesterol and normalize blood pressure. Like other supplements and unlike drugs, the results from alfalfa supplementation take a month before any results are noticed. I think a person has to be really in tune with their body to notice improvements from food supplementation, as improvement is subtle in contrast to drugs. However, the mineral and energy absorption from the far infrared mineral lamp is noticeable immediately as one can get pain relief after a twenty-minute session.

As previously mentioned, research has shown that vitamins cannot be assimilated without the aid of minerals. It is my understanding that the human body can manufacture some vitamins but cannot manufacture any minerals, and yet minerals are essential to our overall mental, emotional, and physical health. Minerals are catalysts for biological functions including muscle response, proper nervous system functioning, hormone production, digestion, and food absorption.

There was a period of my life shortly after my car accident when I had severe cramps and spasms in my legs. The massage therapist suggested that I take more calcium and/or magnesium supplements. Because I was somewhat immobilized as a result of the injury, I think lack of exercise played an important role in my not maintaining the proper calcium content in the body. I can also remember as a student in school being encouraged to drink milk to get the necessary calcium for strong bones and teeth. However, I think there is a major controversy today whether or not the calcium in homogenized milk is absorbable by the body—hence another reason I use the far infrared mineral lamp frequently.

As mentioned previously, I find it helpful to take three or four tablets of calcium and magnesium when I cannot sleep at night. Calcium has so many body functions—maintains proper nerve and muscle activity, lowers blood pressure and blood cholesterol levels, important for proper kidney function, helps regulate the passage of nutrients in and out of the cell walls. I read the other day where some professionals and nutritionists think it may reduce colon cancer. There are many forms of calcium on the market. I like the chewable form—it has a mint flavor, and I feel that by chewing it and mixing it with saliva, it will be absorbed well.

Previously I referred to the concept of the human body surviving for a limited time on minerals and water. My oriental medical doctor often referred to himself as being more energy than matter. He ate very little food, and the little he did eat was low-processed food such as fresh fruit, raw nuts and seeds, and whole grain breads. He was continuously exposed to the far infrared mineral lamp while he worked on clients and drank a goodly amount of chemical-free water. He looked healthy, and it was apparent his body was getting energy it needed from a source other than food. Since he was eating so little, I concluded that the far infrared mineral lamp provided the energy his body needed to run smoothly or he was able to absorb energy from the people he worked on.

In my research on minerals, I learned that in order for minerals to be absorbed efficiently they have to be in a form where they are easily dissolved. One form is chelation, a process in which minerals are combined with something else to increase the utilization rate. Another form is a supplement that is processed at a low temperature and still contains all the other elements found in nature that allow it to be absorbed more easily. It is important that a vitamin supplement not only contains vitamins, but minerals in a form that can be adsorbed by the body, along with other trace minerals. Sometimes I just forego the pill-taking process and rely on obtaining my required minerals from the far infrared mineral lamp. The second and third generation lamps are supposed to have more mineral bars added.

Holistic doctors have treated me with magnesium for many years. I have taken it intravenously with other nutrients. The body needs it to regulate the heart's neuromuscular activity and normal heart rhythm. Sufficient amounts are necessary for calcium & Vitamin C metabolism. I always take calcium with magnesium together in a chewable form. Some symptoms that are a result of a deficiency in calcium are shown to be heart spasms, nervousness, muscular excitability and kidney stones. Several years ago, I developed the most excruciating pain in my left side. I was rushed to the emergency room of the local hospital. They kept me overnight. After taking numerous tests, they concluded the pain was caused by kidney stones. They gave me some equipment to strain my urine in for the next twenty-four hours and sent me home. Sure enough, a few hours later I observed the small black particles from a disintegrated kidney stone. When I saw my naturopathic friend a few days later, he reminded me to take plenty of Vitamin C and magnesium. He also gave me some oriental corn silk to boil and drink as a tea.

Many people in the United States suffer with migraine headaches. Magnesium and calcium therapy works for many people as some research has found lower levels of calcium in the body during a migraine attack.

Iodine aids in the development and proper functioning of the thyroid gland. It is very difficult for doctors to find a way to supplement a patient with this mineral. Iodine helps regulate production of energy and burns excess fat. A deficiency can be noticed in the condition of the hair, skin, and teeth. Deficiency symptoms can be enlarged thyroid gland, but my symptoms were subtler like slow mental reaction, dry skin and hair, weight gain, and loss of physical and mental vigor.

In our country, iodine has been added to salt for many years and so iodine deficiencies are not a major concern. However, some people do not use iodized salt so it is necessary for them to supplement with iodine. It is believed that many of the people being treated with thyroid hormone could get by with supplementing iodine. Originally the doctors told me that I would have to take synthetic thyroid the rest of my life. I use mineral supplementation instead. The problem with supplementation, especially taking B6 for hypothyroidism is that the body adapts to whatever amount is supplemented. Therefore, to maintain normal thyroid function, the supplemented amounts must always be increased, raising the magnesium to high levels. I believe these side effects will not be found by using the far infrared mineral lamp for mineral supplementation.

I was saddened yesterday when I read an article declaring iodine deficiencies a world epidemic as it is estimated that fifty million children were born in 2001 with mental and physical problems. These iodine deficiencies are especially a problem for children living in Pakistan. Mental retardation, due to iodine deficiency in fetal development, is the most serious problem of iodine deficiency.

Potassium iodide is a salt similar to table salt. It is added to table salt to make it iodized. I recently read an article regarding the implementation of potassium iodide in emergency storage for treatment of radiation exposure. The article went on to state that if the proper dosage is taken in time, it can block the uptake of radioactive iodine by the thyroid gland and reduce the effects of thyroid cancer from exposure to radioactive iodine. This is a good thing to stock in emergency storage for protection to treat the effects of radiation exposure caused from damage to a nuclear power plant. Our government has gathered a lot of information from the nuclear exposure at Chernobyl and released documents that can be used for guidance in using potassium iodide as a thyroid-blocking agent in radiation emergencies. I think we live in perilous times and the more educated and responsible each of us can become the stronger we will be as a nation. Potassium iodide has been approved as an over the counter medication. Of course, there is also a problem of overexposure to potassium iodide, so the same precautions that are exercised with other drugs should be applied to the storage of it—keep it out of the reach of children and follow the directions for usage.

I learned that zinc is an antioxidant and is necessary for protein synthesis and wound healing. It is another mineral that I have been deficient in at times in my life, along with many other people because of our depleted soil. My alternative doctor prescribed zinc supplementation for me when I was first diagnosed with breast cancer because it is involved in many enzyme functions and is necessary in building up the immune system and in the detoxification of chemicals. Zinc is used often in the treatment of skin disorders. It can be found in whole grains, but most of it is loss in refined flours. Many things interfere with zinc absorption in the body. I learned a few days ago that the consumption of milk and eggs reduce the absorption of zinc. Stress depletes the body of this mineral.

If trace minerals are taken in excess or in an incompatible ratio to other elements, they can cause problems as well as a deficiency of a specific mineral. During my childbearing years, I suffered with bone spurs in my feet. The foot therapist used ultra sound to treat them. I learned that calcification might not be the result of a high level of calcium but the result of calcium being too high in ratio to other interactive elements. Because calcification had occurred more in my right foot than in my left foot, I learned that it was probably the result of a manganese or magnesium deficiency in the ratio to calcium. If the calcification had been on my left foot, it would probably be the result of a deficiency of phosphorus and zinc in the ratio to calcium. If I had increased my phosphorus and zinc intake, my situation probably would have worsened. The best ratio of trace minerals is the ratio as found in natural food products—nature always knows the correct amount.

Tin and iodine work together in supporting body functions—tin supports the adrenals and iodine supports the thyroid—the thyroid and adrenals interact with cardiac functions—the level of each element can affect the heart function. Other minerals and elements that can affect the thyroid and adrenals are potassium, zinc, manganese, iron, cobalt, nickel, bismuth, lithium, most of the B vitamins, and amino acids. Fatigue and/or depression are symptoms of cardiac insufficiency, but symptoms associated more with deficiencies in the right side of the body are edema and swelling of hands and feet. Because mineral supplementation needs to be in the right ratio, it is important to have a doctor familiar with these ratios prescribe the amount to be taken or use the far infrared mineral lamp like I do because I feel my body will just take the mineral energy it needs and the rest will pass through me.

Several years ago I put myself under the care of a naturopathic doctor who used food to treat diseases. Nutrition can be as effective as antibiotics and other drugs in treating ordinary problems such as urinary, eye, and throat infections. For my liver and kidney problems, he urged me to eat more artichokes and asparagus.

One of the major benefits of using the far infrared mineral lamp is that one does not have to worry about having the right combination of nutrients for efficient absorption because the energy is already in a usable form. It was originally discovered because factory workers of all ages in a China ceramic factory stood in a black clay daily without ever having any arthritic symptoms. Research revealed the clay contained elements and/or minerals with special healing qualities with the same bio-spectrum as the human body and were absorbed by their bodies and used in biological functions.

I have not seen a list of the thirty-three minerals contained in the far infrared mineral lamp. However, others claim that some of the trace minerals are iron, selenium, manganese, zinc, cobalt, nickel, copper, and potassium. Minerals are sometimes referred to as "rocks" because they sometimes enter the body in an unusable form. It is my understanding that the far infrared mineral lamp produces an ionizing effect on these rocks, transforming them into usable energy within the body.

9

Broken Bones and FIR Mineral Therapy

For many years I was a single parent raising five daughters and so poor that all I could afford to drive were old cars—some of them retrieved from junkyards. Finally, my children were all grown and out on their own, and I bought a new car! It was a pretty red Ford Contour with electric windows and many other nice accessories. I had just finished eighteen months of alternative cancer therapies, paying for most of it myself, as it is difficult to get insurance companies to pay for this type of treatment. My co-worker said, "You remind me of a friend of mine who had a dog he adored. The dog was well groomed and lived like royalty. One day the friend was driving down the road with the dog in the back of his pickup when they passed another vehicle with an attractive female dog. The meticulously groomed and expensive dog jumped out of the truck to chase after the car with the female dog. Another car came along and hit the dog. It died immediately!" His owner was very saddened that he had not only lost his best friend, but also a large financial investment in the dog!"

She said, "Kara, I hope that you do not get hurt or killed right away in a car accident after spending all that money on your body." I have often wondered if she had a premonition of things to come—she always told me she could see the aura around my body—maybe her third eye was much more advanced than she was aware of. Because shortly after that, I was on my way to work one morning when I took an alternative route to get gas. It was raining hard, and I was only a few blocks from work when a pickup truck, going the opposite direction, pulled out of the university on the other side of the street. The driver did not see the fast moving car coming up behind him. The pickup hit the car and knocked it over the divider in front of me. I tried to veer right but it all happened too fast, and I hit the car head on and knocked it back over the divider, heading the wrong direction in that lane. We were all pretty lucky. I was knocked out briefly. When

I came to the car was still moving, but on the curb. I put the emergency brake on. Both of the air bags had gone off, my glasses were in the back seat, the hood was all crunched up, and steam was coming out of the engine.

I opened the door and went to step out of the car. Excruciating pain shot up my leg from my left foot. I could not stand on it. The driver of the pickup truck came over and asked me if I was all right. I told him, "I think so but look what has happened to my pretty red car!" I had driven the old clunkers for years and never was in an accident. I drove this nice car for less than eight months, and it was totaled.

I found that I could not put any weight on my left foot. The police arrived and helped me move over to a safe place to sit while I waited for the ambulance. The driver of the pickup was not hurt at all. The passenger in the other car had a broken arm, and the driver had whiplash. In a few minutes the ambulance came. They packed us all into one ambulance and took us to a hospital a few blocks away.

X-rays showed no broken bones in my left foot. However, because of the excruciating pain, the doctor felt there were broken bones in the foot. They ordered an MRI, and found that I had two broken bones in my foot and a dislocated bone. My chest and arms were bruised from the seat belts. They put my foot in a cast and referred me to an orthopedic doctor. I was given instructions to make an appointment to see him in a week. It is customary to place a cast around a broken bone soon after injury. The cast was padded with cotton and wrapped in ace bandages to make it comfortable. The reason plaster was used immediately after my injury is because the plaster casts can be easily fitted to allow for swelling of my foot beneath the cast. Otherwise, the swelling could impair my circulation in my leg and cause more problems. The drawback to using plaster is that it was heavy and cumbersome. I had to keep it dry, which eliminated my using the bathtub for bathing.

It was very hard for me to get around in a cast. That night I almost fell into the bathtub when I was trying to get to the toilet. The doctor had given me prescriptions for painkillers. Prescription drugs are so expensive, and I do not like to take drugs. I decided not to get the prescriptions filled. Besides, the process of getting my health insurance to cover the prescription is complex and bothersome. A friend of mine picked me up, and we drove across the street to a medical device store. I picked up a walker. I already had crutches at home, left over from my daughter's sports days.

That evening I took only two Advil tablets. I wanted so badly to take off the cast and use the far infrared mineral lamp on my foot. I suspected that the lamp might heal my foot much faster and better that the course I was taking. I had four toes sticking out of the cast. I turned the far infrared mineral lamp on and directed it at those four toes. After applying the lamp for twenty minutes, the pain was gone, and I was relaxed. I soon fell asleep and slept all night. I called the OMD the next morning. He was far away in some other state. I asked him, "How can I use the far infrared mineral lamp if I only have four bare toes on that foot to direct it to? He said the healing qualities of the lamp would be absorbed from the exposed toes and have a healing effect on the injured parts covered by the cast. The energy guru also advised me that I could direct the lamp at my other foot and derive the same healing effect on the injured foot. He explained, "Heating one area of the body produces reflex-modulated vasodilatation in distant-body areas, even in the absence of a change in core body temperature. Heat one foot and the other foot also dilates. Heat a forearm and both lower extremities dilate. Heat the front of the trunk and the hand will dilate."

I was really impressed! When I got off the phone with him I applied the lamp to my uninjured foot and could feel the energy moving in the other foot. I contacted my attorney. Because of the legal issues involved, I was advised to be careful and not go overboard on the treatment issues. I confided that I wanted to use the lamp to heal my foot. He advised me to follow the medical doctor's directions, as I would probably end up in court and needed the "medical authority" for standard care treatments. I hated the cast on my foot but I followed my attorney's guidelines.

Finally, the week was up, and I went to see the orthopedic surgeon. He recommended surgery. He wanted to put pins in my foot, fuse the broken bones together, and adjust the dislocated bone. It would take my foot a minimum of ninety days to recover. I did not want surgery and general anesthesia. I did not want to go to a hospital, and I did not want immobilized for three months. I asked, "What are my options?" He said, "You have no options. If you do not have surgery, arthritis will set in and you will eventually be crippled." He wanted to do the surgery the next day—I told him I needed time to think about it. He then told me he would need to put the cast back on my foot if I was not going to have surgery the following day.

While he was preparing the cast room, I borrowed my friends cell phone and called an orthopedic medical doctor who used medicine to treat broken bones, not surgery. I was fortunate that there was a cancellation the very next morning. I made the appointment and told the doctor not to put the cast on as I was going to get a second opinion. The doctor gave me a prescription for a wheel chair. My friend and I picked up the wheel chair before heading home.

I arrived at the alternative doctor's office in the wheelchair the following morning. The doctor was surprised and asked me what I was doing in the wheelchair. I told him the orthopedic surgeon prescribed the wheelchair. He told me I had no business in the wheelchair, as I needed to be using the foot to prevent more swelling. My foot was swelled up like a balloon because it had not been used for a week! I was confused—I thought my foot was in a cast to control the swelling.

The doctor did a complete examination. Neither the hospital emergency room nor the orthopedic surgeon had done a complete examination. The examination revealed that my right knee was also injured in the car accident. He asked, "Did the other doctors note that the knee was injured?' I said, "No!"

The doctor told me it was too late to do a closed reduction (the reduction of a displaced part by manipulation without incision). It would have had to be done in twenty-four hours following the injury. "However, he said, "You do have options other than surgery." He said, "Prolotherapy is very effective on this type of injury."

He explained that prolotherapy is the treatment of soft-tissue damage through the use of an injection of a proliferant, which leads to inflammation in the area. The doctor demonstrated that the pain in my injured foot was due to the swelling and bruised soft tissues, not the broken bone. He said, "The induced inflammation increases the blood supply and sends more nutrients to the area, resulting in tissue repair.

The idea behind prolotherapy dates back more than two thousand years. I read where Hippocrates used it to treat soldiers. Prolotherapy has been used to treat varicose veins, chronic neck pain, arthritis, headache, fibromyalgia, sports injuries, and carpal tunnel syndrome. This is a non-surgical procedure that was going to be performed in the doctor's office, saving me from undergoing general anesthesia, surgery, and a long recovery period. It is much cheaper than surgery. Washington law requires a person's PIP insurance to pay for medical care and then be reimbursed by the responsible insurance company upon claim settlement. I only had $10,000 of PIP insurance and felt that I could not afford surgery, anesthesia, hospital cost, and physical therapy, which would have been approximately $30,000. The doctor assured me that there would be no loss of mobility with prolotherapy in contrast to the surgery, and I would not have the highly marked-up cost and side effects of prescription painkillers.

The proliferant consists of sugar or salt water-based solution injected into the damaged ligaments and tendons at the point where it attaches to the bone, causing the body to think it has another injury and start the repair and healing process.

I agreed to the prolotherapy. The doctor said that before he could do prolotherapy, it would be necessary to apply lymphatic massage in an effort to push the fluid up my leg. The swelling decreased after several days of lymphatic massage. The prolotherapy treatment was then used on my foot. Two weeks after the accident, I was back at work, walking on my foot. I elevated my foot as much as possible while sitting at my desk. The doctor explained to me that exercise and use would be beneficial and very important to the healing process of my injured foot.

Because of the legal issues that were involved in the three-car accident, my attorney advised me it was imperative that licensed medical doctors treat me. I believed that I could have used the far infrared mineral lamp on my foot twice a day for forty minutes and received healing faster and less cumbersome than either of the other treatment processes suggested by the doctors. I have faith and confidence that the far infrared mineral lamp would have emitted energy my body could use to affect the same self-healing that the proliferant did. However, I am grateful that the alternative medical doctor had the prolotherapy knowledge and skills, saving me from drugs and surgery.

I recently read an article by an oriental medical doctor who wrote that there are numerous bone fracture cases on record where the bones had not healed properly years after the original treatment. He further stated that a far infrared mineral lamp has the capability to heal these fracture in less than two years. He stated that zinc, one of the thirty-three elements in the black plate, is essential for the body to convert proteins, and that regular usage of the far infrared mineral lamp would attract and activate protein function. In addition, to activating the protein function, the lamp emits special energy to stimulate and increase bone cell growth rate by increasing calcium and phosphorus for transfer to bone fracture ending. This process accelerates bone healing.

I know several oriental medical doctors in close proximity to where I live that are familiar with the far infrared mineral therapy lamp and know how to use it to treat a broken foot. It is unfortunate that we are so regulated that sometimes freedom of choice is overridden by the need to conform to laws and/or consensus of popular opinion.

10

Work-Related Injuries

For several years I was safety director for a small manufacturing company. Because of the fine detail work performed under a microscope, there was a problem with work-related injuries caused by the employees having to sit in a static position while peering through a microscope and using their hands and fingers to do fine detail work.

The partial fix or cure for reducing the number of work-related injuries was the implementation and conversion to ergonomic equipment and implementing mini breaks with many short, fast paced walks to increase the circulation. Carpal tunnel and tendonitis were common work-related musculoskeletal injuries as a result of this type of employment.

After months of speculation and congressional questioning, OSHA has finally released its plan to reduce these types of injuries. There has been much controversy over whether or not the employer is as fault in these issues or if it is deficiencies in the individual that is responsible. OSHA's new plan stresses voluntary compliance—the mandatory regulation was killed by the republican-controlled congress in 2001. Based on my personal experiences, both as the injured and as a safety director, I believe that these types of injuries have more to do with the lifestyles of an employee than on the working conditions at a company. Even after switching to full ergonomics, I found that these types of injuries still occurred in individuals with lifestyles characterized by substance abuse, inactivity, poor eating habits, and stress from personal problems. Emotional stress appeared to be the most prevalent in all of the cases.

Part of the new OSHA program will be producing industry and task-specific guidelines to provide the best practices for reducing ergonomic injuries in high-risk industries. Many of these industries employ Hispanic and other immigrant workers. This program will cost the government and corporations a lot of money, as it will require not only equipment conversion, but also education. Like all government programs, there will be a lot of grant money for research.

Several weeks ago I developed tendonitis in my biceps as a result of inputting a lot of computer data. I had been living a sedentary lifestyle, not eating properly, and dealing with a lot of emotional stress. In addition, I did not have an ergonomic workstation. Ergonomic workstations are a great help in preventing work-related injuries from repetitive movements, but are very costly for the employer to implement.

Some principles of ergonomics are as follows: The chair is the starting place in applying ergonomics. The chair should have good back support and the chair height should be adjustable to a comfortable height for me. Armrest design is important and should be movable and adjustable so that the elbows do not rest in one place for long periods of time. A desk designed for writing is often too high for typing. The keyboard should be about the same height or slightly lower than the elbow.

The first step taken by conventional medicine to treat such an injury as mine is usually to apply cold packs to the injured area. When an injury or inflammation such as tendonitis occurs, tissues are damaged. The application of cold packs numbs the affected area, reducing pain, tenderness, swelling, and inflammation. Most conventional teachings suggest cold pack applications for these types of injuries. However, the OMD suggested only using cold packs initially on these types of injuries, and using follow up applications of heat because heat brings more blood to the area reducing joint stiffness and muscle spasm. Heat helps to resolve inflammation and eliminate chemical side products (toxins) produced from the exercise and use of muscles. When muscles are overused or after intense exercise, there may not be enough blood flow to eliminate all of the toxins. It is the accumulation of toxins such as lactic acid that causes muscle ache and pain. Heat can be an important application in these types of injuries. Sometimes it is confusing whether to use heat or cold when treating sore muscles or injuries.

There are several types of warm packs and/or pads. One type is wetting a towel with hot water and applying it to the affected area. Another type is using a heating pad. Care should be given to avoid burns by not putting a heating pad device in direct contact with the skin.

There are several ways of making cold packs and/or pads. One method is to wet a towel with cold water, fold it, and insert it is a sealed plastic bag, and then place the plastic bag in the freezer for fifteen minutes or so. Another method is to place ice in the bag, partially fill it with water, seal the bag, and apply to the affected area. Preparing and applying hot and cold packs are time consuming!

Over the counter painkillers are sometimes prescribed by doctors to treat this type of injury. Sometimes the doctor will prescribe physical therapy. After applying the hot or cold packs, sometime a physical therapist will apply cortisone cream and use ultra sound to help the absorption of the cream into the injured area. A physician often prescribes bandages and splints—careful attention needs to be given because they can restrict blood flow, making the symptoms worse.

Often the physician will restrict the use of the hand or limb until the hand is healed.

I have tried to present an image of how time consuming and costly the treatment of these types of injuries can be. I found that the far infrared mineral lamp simplifies the treatment and great reduces the healing time and cost of therapy. In addition, there is little, if any, loss of time.

In this particular instance, I was not aware of the inflammation and/or tendonitis in my biceps until the morning after the overuse. I used the far infrared mineral lamp on my bicep and shoulder for approximately twenty minutes before going to work. I noticed some relief in the pain and soreness, but it was still painful to raise my arm. I went to work and soon forgot about the injury when I became involved in critical issues. By mid-afternoon, I noticed that the pain and soreness was gone from my arm, and that I could easily raise and lower it without the previous pain and discomfort.

The far infrared mineral lamp accomplished all of the affects of the foregoing conventional therapies and complete healing occurred within a matter of hours. The lamp increased the blood supply to the area, allowing toxins (lactic acid, etc.) to be removed from the affected area. The absorbable mineral energy emitted by the black mineral plate of the lamp brought usable energy to the area allowing self-healing to take place immediately and quickly.

I do not believe there is any other sports injury or work-related musculoskeletal injury therapy that has the immediate and quick healing capabilities of the far infrared mineral lamp. Because it is a new concept, its acceptance by conventional medicine, especially OSHA and the Department of Labor & Industries (workman's compensation) may be slow due to the usual opposition to an alternative-healing concept regardless of the fact that the lamp has already been approved by the FDA.

The lamp has been highly successful in treating thousands of soft tissue injuries as a result of sports, accidental trauma, and spinal injuries. One of the major benefits is its ability to quickly and effectively decrease inflammation and edema resulting from these types of injuries. The far infrared mineral lamp has been used in China for sports related injuries since 1984.

Far infrared mineral therapy is very effective in treating bruises and hematoma. Based on my own experiences, generally ninety per cent of the pain, swelling, and discoloration will be eliminated after two treatments and one day.

My youngest daughter played basketball and other sports in high school. She has had one surgical operation on her ankles and has been recommend for another surgery. The ligaments in her ankles are stretched, and she can do contortionist movements with her foot. Even though the injuries occurred six years ago, I encourage her to use the far infrared mineral lamp on her ankles, because I believe she can attain miraculous healing these many years after the injury by using the lamp. I have heard testimonies from others who have successfully used the lamp two times a week for twenty to forty minutes for three months to eliminate pain.

I read about another case where a man incurred a head injury leaving him paralyzed on one side of his body, unable to speak audibly, and walk without difficulty. With regular application of far infrared mineral therapy eighteen months later, both speech and body movement improved considerably. In China, the lamp has been proven effective in the treatment of other neurological disorders such as migraine and sciatica.

Some people I know use the lamp regularly each day for various aches and pains. Some use it just to feel better. I use it for both reasons.

11

Anti-Aging Remedies

Americans live longer than ever before. There is an increasing interest in anti-aging medicine. ABC recently had a news release on a village in Japan where ten percent of the residents lived to be eighty-five and older, still farming and leading other high quality lives without showing the signs of aging. The local diet is attributed with providing the elements for this ageless living in rare foods such as satsumaimo, a sweet potato, satoimo, a white potato, and imoji, a potato root. Since these all belong to the family of root vegetables, it brings to my mind what an old naturopathic once told a sickly friend of mind, "You are not eating enough root vegetables." It is believed that these locally grown, starchy vegetables contain elements that help stimulate the body's natural creation of a substance called hyaluornic acid, (HA).

Hyaluornic acid is essential for the proper functioning of joints. As we age the level of joint fluid decreases and changes causing the cartilage to break down resulting in osteoarthritis. Hyaluornic acid supplements are sold in health food stores.

Russia has its own theory on aging. Russian scientific research shows that aging is not caused by the passing of years, but by an overload of information stored at a cellular level in the body. Based on this evidence, they believe that the only treatment that can be called anti-aging is the one that allows the body to reduce the level of unnecessary information in cellular memory. Their product, Alozone-M, is believed to accelerate anticancer action of radiation therapy and protect normal tissue from the harmful action of radiation, making the immune system stronger.

In America, there are many anti-aging remedies on the market. One is a product called HGH Revolution that is packaged, as an easy to use oral spray comprised of one hundred ninety-one amino acids. Cognitive Factors is another one that provides advanced support for cognitive function, helping with mild memory problems associated with aging.

Throughout the ages, people have tried to find the fountain of youth. Today is no different. Is there a fountain of youth? Well, the closest I have found is the far infrared mineral lamp. Some people claim that effects of sunlight can be similar to physical exercise because it can increase the oxygen level in cells, muscle strength, and vitality. Sunlight can provide mental stability as evidenced in the Northwest by the increase in depression during the rainy season. Some health care professionals believe that sunlight helps regulate hormonal activity, enhance immune function, and facilitate bone growth.

As I begin to age, I experienced menopause, fatigue, and insomnia. As I mentioned earlier, the far infrared mineral lamp helps me sleep when I am experiencing insomnia. I believe the bio-spectrum energy emitted from the lamp may be beneficial and helpful in reversing the degenerative effects of aging. This bio-spectrum energy may be essential to the proper functioning of the endocrine system. I have never used synthetic estrogen hormone replacement. However, I feel that using the far infrared mineral lamp may be a much safer and more effective way of maintaining proper hormone functioning.

In previous chapters I have discussed some of the degenerative processes that I have experienced growing older such as digestive problems and osteoarthritis. Other people my age often experience hypertension, osteoporosis, and headaches due to over acidity. In my book, *Breast Cancer: Death Call or Enlightenment,* I discuss the importance of alkalizing the body to prevent the degenerative process. Americans love acid-forming foods such as animal meat, highly processed foods, and fast food restaurants. I believe that far infrared mineral lamp therapy may help eliminate this aging process because of the mineral absorption and the increased body heat caused by the infrared resonance that increases the blood circulation. This increased body heat may help in removing acidic build-up in the arteries.

The far infrared mineral lamp bio-spectrum energy is believed by some to contain negative ions that help reverse the aging process. Several years ago when I was experiencing many environmental sensitivity problems, I used an ionizer to clean the air in my apartment and especially in my bedroom. The increase in the negative ions made me more comfortable, more relaxed and happier due to the increase in serotonin in my bloodstream. Recent research has shown negative ions may be effective in preventing infections and migraines.

I live in the foothills of the Cascade Mountains and have been told that the Chinook winds that blow through the Cascades from Canada contain large amounts of negative ions. Every time the wind starts blowing, I tell myself that the winds are bringing me good health. Negative ions can be found near the ocean and waterfalls. One of my favorite places is the ocean where I can breathe deeper and feel energized from the ocean air. When the Snoqualmie Valley River rises, I love to go to the Snoqualmie Falls and inhale the rich negative ions from the gushing water over the falls.

Most of the rest of our environment is lacking in negative ions due to the way our houses are built—concrete and plastics in our infrastructure and buildings. These materials absorb the negative ions from the atmosphere. The one man-made structure that may increase negative ions is the shower—the falling water may create negative ions.

Far infrared appears to me to be the best technology for breaking up and neutralizing toxins in the body. As mentioned in earlier chapters, the warming effect of far infrared stimulates metabolism and blood circulation, bringing nutrients and oxygen to soft tissue. It also stimulates the lymphatic process, enhancing the removal of toxins and acids. It was my interest in detoxifying that first led me to the far infrared mineral lamp. Today far infrared is becoming the cutting edge technology in detoxification. Infrared saunas are believed to yield many health benefits—relief from pain, enhanced immune function, improved skin, and accelerated burning of calories. The infrared sauna promotes detoxification through the sweat process.

Ionized water filters and drops also are used to help alkalize the body. Ionized alkaline water is a new water purification approach. The promoters of ionized alkaline water believe it to have anti-aging and reverse aging benefits because aging is caused by dehydration and an accumulation of acid waste resulting in disease. As I have stated previously, one of the first things the OMD told me was that I was not drinking enough water. He encouraged me to drink at least a gallon of clean, purified water daily as hydration and detoxification reverse the aging process.

Ionizer water filters create ionized alkaline water through a process called electrolysis to raise the pH to a more alkaline level. Ionized water has antioxidant properties that are believed to counteract free radical *damage*.

Another contributor to the aging process is believed to be the decline in the earth's natural magnetic field. The same culprits that absorb the negative ions are responsible for the decline in the earth's magnetism—concrete roadways, steel buildings, and automobiles. As mentioned earlier, science has determined that there is a relationship between the earth's magnetic field and the human body's magnetic field. Some believe the earth's decreased magnetic field causes imbalances in the human body. The electric appliances we use in our home emit low frequency currents that lower our natural biorhythms. More information on the affects of electricity on health can be found in Robert O. Becker's book, *Cross Currents: The Promise of Electromedicine, the Perils of Electropollution.*

I have a friend whose mother has lived in a nursing home since she was fifty years old. Today she is sixty-five. It was hard for me to understand why someone would make this kind of a decision since some of the best years of my life occurred during these years. My daughter has a friend who was a young male only twenty-four years old who has aged very rapidly. He has spent a good deal of his life on prescription drugs, fast food, cigarettes, substance abuse, and not drinking enough water.

There are many different theories on how to reverse the aging process. Sang Whang discusses reversing the aging process using ionized water more fully in his book, *Reverse Aging.* Sang Wang is a scientist, engineer, and inventor. The improvement in his own health initiated his writing this book.

I believe that regular use of the far infrared mineral lamp is one of the best anti-aging remedies available to day as the human body can absorb the full spectrum mineral energy that the body needs to ionize minerals and use them, slowing down the aging process.

I, along with everybody else, require a continuous supply of far infrared (FIR) from the sun to boost the powers of FIR found in our bodies. Adequate exposure to sunlight helps us feel more energetic and healthier. It is my understanding that when FIR comes in contact with my body, which has a similar resonance causing them both to vibrate at the same frequency, FIR is absorbed and forms a natural energy and heat. It is believed that when the FIR in our bodies starts to decline, we develop illnesses and diseases, grow old, and eventually die.

I believe that regular use of the far infrared mineral lamp is one of the best anti-aging remedies available to day as the human body can absorb the full spectrum mineral energy that the body needs to ionize minerals and use them, slowing down the aging process. FIR is able to penetrate deep in the body, activating cells, regulating blood flow by breaking up blood clots, and reactivating Qi, our vital energy.

I believe the far infrared mineral lamp increases our metabolism. When nutrients are absorbed from the food we eat, waste products are produced and need to be removed from the body. By improving the blood circulation, FIR increases the metabolic rate, increasing energy and vitality, which builds up immunity against diseases.

The end result may be increased longevity!

12

Stress, Worry, and Negative Emotions

I consider myself as having been a caregiver for most of my life. I have never been able to not try to solve my children's problems (and other people problems). Consequently, I am never fully prepared to deal with everybody else's problems and end up emotionally drained after trying to find resolution. Many times I find myself consumed with fear, anxiety, frustration, depression, anger, and irritability because I become overwhelmed with all of these emotional challenges.

I do not do a very good job of dealing with emotions. I guess I am one of those people who never learned to throw things when frustrated, or scream and kick—I keep my feelings repressed, and they show up in my spine as spinal misalignments (sublaxations). My network chiropractor and other energy gurus have told me that my needs were not met while I was carried in my mother's womb and in the first year of my life. It is during this period of our life that we begin to develop our emotions.

I have spent the last two and one-half years seeing a network chiropractor. With the application of network spinal analysis most of the distortions are gone from my spine. However, integration is a slow process. Network Spinal Analysis (NSA) is a new approach to wellness using light touch to the spine and surrounding tissues to help the brain connect with the rest of the body. Somato Respiratory Integration (SRI) is a self-help technique taught by my chiropractor and a means of establishing connections between the brain and the rest of the body through innate intelligence with the use of various exercises of touch and breathing. Donald M. Epstein, D.C, developed both NSA and SRI and has written books on these techniques—T*he Twelve Stages of Healing* and *Healing Myths, Healing Magic.*

In the book, *The Twelve Stages of Healing,* Dr. Epstein describes the complex healing relationship between mind, emotions, and the physical body. He portrays how each stage of healing has a healing crisis that helps us reunite with trauma-tized, alienated, forgotten, abused, shamed or unforgiving aspects of ourselves. He shows how each stage of healing has a characteristic pattern of breath, move-ment, and touch that helps us connect with the natural, internal rhythms of our body, enabling us to experience a greater sense of well-being. I recently visited one of my daughters in Michigan who was expecting her second baby. Prior to my trip departure, the visit to my network chiropractor revealed that a shift in my energy field was about to take place.

The day before my return trip home, I experienced profuse releases of bile and mucous which continued on my return flight home. In addition to the awkward trips to the tiny toilet in a Boeing 737 plane filled to capacity, I found myself experiencing anger and uncontrollable crying. When I saw my network chiro-practor the following day, he observed new shifts in my energy field. When I con-fided to him my concerns about the profuse releases of bile and mucous, he suggested that my body might be discharging information that it no longer needed.

If I had not already experienced these types of releases before and looked to the conventional medical doctor for advice and diagnosis instead of my holistic doctor, my conventional medical doctor probably would have ordered numerous costly diagnostic tests and drugs, and may have even ordered exploratory surgery. Is it any wonder that health care expense is so high in the United States? Several days have passed and so have these symptoms. My stools are again normal, and I have no pain, anger, or tears.

As I said previously, integration is a slow process with me because of the many emotional issues in my life. I have tried to get by with seeing my network chiro-practor less often than once a week. Without the weekly adjustments, life is more difficult.

I have found the far infrared mineral lamp to be very helpful between chiro-practic visits, especially in providing comfort and easing the pain in my lower back and in the muscles around my rib cage.

A short time ago, I entered my network chiropractor's office with lower back pain and pressure, making it difficult for me to stand for extended periods of time. I reflected upon how I may have gotten my self into such a dilapidated con-dition. I concluded that I had been working in a very stressful situation for quite awhile. First, the ventilation in the office was not good, contaminated with recy-cled cigarette smoke and various chemicals such as formaldehyde from the storage of corrugated boxes. At the same time, the company was going through difficult times—its longevity was questionable. There were many ways I could have dealt with the stress differently—but I chose to deal with it as I have always done—by not dealing with it. When I finally left the place, I practically had to crawl into my chiropractor's office for a treatment. I left his office with more energy and greater flexibility.

I was able to increase the length between my visits to the network chiropractor by using the far infrared mineral lamp twice a day. By applying it to the tight muscles in my lower back, I am able to alleviate the pain for short intervals. It never occurred to me to apply it to my upper neck, which is where the problem was originating—I only applied it to where I felt the pain—my mid back and rib cage. It is still difficult for me to remember that the pain in my lower back might be due to what is going on in my neck.

As explained in other sections of this book, minerals are essential to human life. It is estimated that as high as four per cent of the entire human body mass is derived from minerals. The spinal fluid contains concentrations of minerals since nerve cells are comprised of minerals that act as catalysts and play a vital role in strengthening skeletal structures and proper functioning of the neurological system.

Many professionals and researchers believe that all of us are mineral deficient in one capacity or another. Mineral deficiencies can be caused by physical or emotional stress, dehydration, poor intestinal absorption, malnutrition, and mineral-deficient foods.

For several months, I was engaged in detoxification processes in an effort to remove emotional and chemical toxins from my body, which my immunologist believed was partly responsible for the malignant tumor in my breast. Some professionals believe that the colonic itself can cause loss of, or an imbalance in, the trace mineral absorption process. I find the far infrared mineral lamp invaluable in helping me restore the minerals in my body caused by the emotional issues and detoxification processes.

I believe that far infrared mineral therapy helps fight stress by promoting body functions to restore and repair damage. Stress plays a role in major health problems—cancer, heart disease, and stroke. By reducing stress in my life through safe and natural far infrared mineral therapy, I hope to experience a longer, quality life.

13

Seasonal Affective Disorder (SAD)

When the seasons change, both animals and humans are affected and change daily habits. Most people eat and sleep more in winter when the sun is hidden a good deal of the time. My dog, Muffin, ate and slept more in the winter. The primary source of energy for all living things is the sun and comes in two forms—light and heat. Heat energy cannot be captured directly by plants, animals, and humans; it does warm up the non-living objects surrounding them. Animals and humans use heat energy to warm up their bodies, but need to eat food to acquire energy for sustaining life. Plants contain an energy-capturing substance called chlorophyll and use a process called photosynthesis to convert light energy into stored energy.

Many people throughout the world suffer from Seasonal Affective Disorder (SAD) sometimes referred to as winter blues. People suffering with SAD or winter blues feel worse between the months of September and April. Incidences of SAD increase all around the world with increased distance from the equator (except where the ground is covered with snow). SAD is attributed to lack of bright light in winter.

I have a twenty-four year old friend who is unable to work and suffers from depression and a myriad of other behavior difficulties. He can sleep twenty-four hours in a row—it is very difficult for him to get out of bed in the morning after a night of insomnia and anxiety. When awakened in the morning he is irritable and mean because he is not refreshed from having a good night's sleep. Because he feels so bad after such a night he avoids company whenever possible. He complains of stomach problems, headaches, flu and similar illnesses, has a hard time coping with ordinary every-day problems. Unable to come up with any disease or physical condition to attribute his discomfort and ailments to, the medical doctors diagnosed him as bipolar and clinical insane. Someone from the Mayo Clinic simplified the definition of bipolar by characterizing the symptoms as "from high to low, from euphoria to depression, and from recklessness to listlessness." Medical doctors estimate that it affects millions of adults in America. It is a serious and disabling mental illness.

After my previous bout with cancer, I have learned to look at my health problems and others' by trying to analyze the whole person and his/her lifestyle. My friend lives in the basement of his grandmother's house a good deal of the time. There are windows, but the rooms are very dark. He smokes cigarettes, drinks coffee on a daily basis, uses alcoholic beverages, dislikes vegetables, and craves the carbohydrates found in processed and fast food. After sleeping most of the day, his late evenings are spent eating, watching movies and television, and smoking more because he cannot sleep.

Based on my own experiences, I have wondered how my friend would respond to light therapy. There are many forms of light therapy—full spectrum overhead lighting in office buildings is one form. In the northwest, skiing is a very popular self-therapy for SAD while others become snowbirds, living in hot places like Arizona during the fall and winter months because they feel better in the warmer climate with more light.

The Chinese consider Qi and bio-spectrum energies of the human body to be very important and their deficiencies and imbalances relative to disease. The far infrared mineral lamp that I use to treat pain and enhance my immune system was developed by the Chinese and approved for use in America by the FDA.

Far Infrared (FIR) cannot be seen. It is an invisible part of the full spectrum of sunlight and is sometimes referred to as the light of life because all life, including plants, animals, and humans, need the FIR found in sunlight to reproduce and develop. The human body produces FIR, similar to that of sunlight. The healing powers of many Qigong masters are a result of strong FIR emissions by their bodies. Some people believe that when the FIR produced by the human begins to decline, degenerative diseases set in, and eventually death occurs. Constant exposure to sunlight is needed to keep the FIR in our bodies at the level needed to remain healthy and delay the aging process.

As the sun's rays began to warm up the earth in early spring, it was customary for my dog, Muffin, to lie in the sun for long periods. I remember a couple of years ago when we experienced an exceptional dreary winter that I found myself reacting the same as my dog when encountering the sun's warmth and sunlight after its absence for several months—I found a bench in a park and spent my lunch hour lying on the bench, absorbing the warmth from the sun's rays. It has been a beautiful fall this year—more sun than usual. My daughter and I were driving in a park. The trees were bursting with all of their beauty—I was mesmerized with the bright reds, yellows, and browns. I vocally told the trees how beautiful I thought they were. I wanted so much to stop the car and find a place where I could stretch out in the sun and consume its warmth and light, but my daughter had an appointment she wanted to keep, and I had to forego experiencing this sensation until another day.

Some people who work in buildings suffer from SAD-type symptoms the year around. They suffer from depression that involves decreased appetite, sleep, and weight loss. Others not only suffer the winter depression, but also have mild and sometimes-severe manic mood swings in the spring and summer. Like my young twenty-four year old friend, they are often diagnosed as Bipolar Disorder. Their symptoms are so severe that often Lithium, a mood stabilizer, is prescribed. The effectiveness of antidepressants in treating depression is a controversial issue as some research has shown that giving a person a placebo that mimics the side effects of the drugs are just as effective.

It is estimated that about seventy percent of people suffering with SAD are women. Why does that not surprise me? There appears to be some connection between SAD symptoms and where a sufferer lives in the world. Some people live summer months in one area and move to warmer, sunnier climates in the winter. For people working in office buildings, they suffer the year around. Others are so sensitive that they experience mood changes each time the weather is cloudy.

I grew up on a farm in Iowa. At the age of seven, my brother and I learned to get up early in the morning, even in winter, to milk cows and do other farm chores before we ate breakfast and left for school. In the evening, we performed the evening farm chores, ate the evening meal, and then retired early shortly after the sun went down. The length of our day was determined by daylight.

As stated in the first chapter, the oriental medical doctor taught that all life—plant, animal, and human—exists in a magnetic field and respond to the magnetic field of the Earth. Animals have definite behavior patterns that are not only influenced by the earth's magnetic field but also by the change of seasons (day/night cycle), which is relative to the changes in the earth's magnetic field.

Humans, like the animals, are influenced by the day/night cycle. The desire to sleep in both is triggered by melatonin, a hormone produced by the pineal gland. When the sun sets in the evening, the decreased level of sunlight initiate's the production of melatonin, which causes drowsiness and a desire to sleep. Morning sunlight, entering through the eye to the pineal gland, halts the melatonin production, terminating the desire to sleep.

Western medicine does not know what causes SAD. The hormone melatonin is the prime suspect because it is believed that people suffering with SAD release more melatonin in the winter months. Another reason may be that SAD sufferers do not sleep more in the winter when the nights are longer.

Some people suspect prescription, nonprescription drugs, and alcohol may be responsible for the onset of SAD, too. If a person is suffering with SAD, it may be a good idea to take an inventory of the drugs being used and analyze their side effects.

Research has shown that many elderly people in nursing homes are deficient in vitamin D because they are confined to indoors. Regular indoor lighting impairs the absorption of calcium in the intestines. Researchers also found that when rats were kept in a windowless room, they attacked each other. John N. Ott reveals a lot of information on the effects of light in his book. *Health and Light: The Effects of Natural and Artificial Light on Man and Other Living Things.*

Light therapy or phototherapy is the most common therapy for SAD. This is usually accomplished through the use of a portable lighting device known as a light box. The patient sits in front of the box for a prescribed period of time ranging from fifteen minutes to a couple of hours. Light therapy is an effective and safe treatment for SAD. However, light therapy may be harmful to people with eye disease—it is a good idea to consult your doctor before using it.

Alternative therapies always look for nutritional deficiencies in any disease or unhealthy condition. With SAD, deficiencies in various vitamins, minerals, and amino acids are recognized as playing an important role—specifically calcium, magnesium, chromium, selenium, iron, and zinc.

As stated earlier in this book, there have been times in my life when I crave the warmth and light from the sun and just want to lie in its rays. I do experience some depression and a decrease in energy when the sun is absent for a good deal of the time in the winter months.

I use the far infrared mineral lamp when I am experiencing any of these SAD-like symptoms. As discussed earlier in this book, the lamp does not have a light bulb—the black mineral plate produces far infrared mineral energy that can be absorbed and used by the human body. Far Infrared (FIR) cannot be seen. It is an invisible part of the full spectrum of sunlight and is sometimes referred to as the light of life because all life, including plants, animals, and humans, need the FIR found in sunlight to remain healthy.

14

Pets and FIR Mineral Lamp Therapy

My dog, Muffin, is no longer with us. I miss her when I open the door, and she is not on the front step, happily greeting me. When I drive in the driveway, I look for her to come bouncing up to the car to greet me like she has done for the previous sixteen years. Then I remember—she is gone! Muffin was part husky and something else. She was black, so I tend to think she must have had some black Labrador in her. Because of her thick, heavy fur she lived outside all of the time, even in snow and freezing weather. She was a hunter—she would get bored with commercial dog feed and go find her own fresh meat. She especially liked pheasant and chicken.

I was a single parent trying to raise three young daughters when Muffin came to live with us. She was a replacement for my daughter's dog, Poopey, who was hit by a car and killed shortly after we moved into our new home. Poopey had been a birthday gift for Kelly, and she served us very well in the short time she was with us. Within days after Poopey came to live with us, she had been willing to sacrifice her life to protect us. We were living in a townhouse in a nearby city. One night around 2:30 a.m., our little pup's barking awakened me. I was confused because I had secured Poopey in a room in the garage before going to bed and now her barking appeared to becoming from the stairwell in our house. On this particular evening, Kelly and I were the only ones home. The other two children were spending the weekend at their father's.

I crept out of bed and started down the stairs. It was wintertime and the house was drafty. I had hung a blanket over the stairwell opening to stop the draft that came from the upper level. Halfway down the stairs, there was a small landing where the stairs turned. I could see Poopey who was only a few steps ahead of me barking at something on the other side of the blanket. Suddenly I stopped and went no further. I was being warned to go back upstairs by an entity from the spirit world that talked to my mind—there were no audible works spoken. I found myself arguing with my thoughts that I had to go downstairs because that was where the phone was. After the entity told me three times to go back upstairs, I did! As I climbed back up the stairs, I was wondering what good I could do by retreating. As I entered my room, I looked out the window and saw two teenage girls leave their house across the street. I opened the window and asked them to call the police because I had intruders in the house.

They retreated back into the house. My young daughter awoke when we heard the phone receiver picked up in the lower level. Subsequently, the girls and their mother came outside and the mother told me she had called the police. She then asked what door they had come in. I told them probably the back door. She started around the apartment complex to look. She later told me that she saw two older teenagers leave through my back gate and run down the alley.

In a few minutes the police arrived with a dog. The dog lost the scent several doors down. I was too scared to move, but finally forced myself to go back down the stairs and let the police in. They told me the small puppy had probably saved our lives, as an older man had been murdered a week previously when thugs broke into his house looking for drugs. I smiled to myself upon reflecting how Poopey had needed help from a spiritual entity in protecting us. Her barking awoke me; however, if my guardian angel or whoever the entity was, had not encouraged me to go back upstairs, we may have all been killed, including Poopey.

Little Poopey was less than six months old when she was hit and killed by a speeding motorist in front of our new house. Shortly thereafter, Muffin came to live with us. As Muffin was an outside dog, we thought she needed company so we found a companion for her, Cupcake. The dogs got along really well. Cupcake was continually finding trouble, and Muffin was continually getting her out of trouble. Muffin was strong and few dogs would try to fight her. Prior to the time that Cupcake came to live with us, Muffin slept in a big hollow tree stump in our bag yard. She looked like a big burly bear as she came out of the stump.

Cupcake found some trouble one day that eventually cost her life. The newspaper person, an older lady, came to our door. Cupcake was not a vicious dog or an aggressive dog. Cupcake softly nipped her pant leg. The newspaper person was not a dog lover. She claimed Cupcake had bitten her and notified the authorities. I was forced to lock her up in a kennel. She barked a lot because she wanted to be out with Muffin. One night, someone threw some poisoned meat into the kennel. She died at the vet's office.

Muffin adjusted to whatever the situation. She was a happy dog. As she grew older, I refused to keep her tied on a leash because I felt she deserved her freedom. She only saw the vet a few times in her long dog life because I did not have the money to do otherwise. Since she lived much longer than the average dog, I have reflected on how this happened when she was deprived of the vet care, grooming, special attention, high priced commercial food, and toys that other pet lovers give their pets. What comes to my mind the most is the fact that she lived outside all the time in natural light, living close to nature, keeping her natural instincts in operation. I believe that pets, like humans, need the benefits of full-spectrum light found in natural sunlight to stay healthy.

When she was about fifteen years old, one of my daughters took her to a vet to have some cysts removed. She was given a prescription to help her incontinence. The drugs were very expensive and after a short time no longer effective. As she aged, she developed arthritis and found it difficult to walk. The poor dog was partially blind and pretty deaf towards the end, but she still defended her turf. I still let Muffin go on walks with me. I believed that, like humans, it is best to keep walking dogs since activity keeps the joints more mobile.

The early signs of canine osteoarthritis are stiffness, limping, lagging behind on walks, and inactivity. Osteoarthritis is one of the most common canine diseases and the most common causes of pain. Usually by the time the disease is noticed, irreparable structural damage to joint cartilage may have already occurred. The disease progresses much more rapidly in dogs than it does in humans.

Dogs, like humans, respond very well to warming a sore joint. The far infrared mineral lamp works wonderfully on these kinds of canine problems. Dogs are comforted by touch and do better if they know that someone cares about them.

For those pets that live inside most of their life and do not have the opportunity Muffin had to live close to nature, there are breathable warm and lightweight pet pads made with far infrared technology that provide natural warmth. The pads are activated by body temperature and have magnets to sooth tired doggy or cat muscles and help the pets become refreshed and energized.

There are several good books on natural pet therapy—*Natural Healing for Dogs and Cats* by Diane Stein and *Natural Health for Dogs and Cats* by Richard H. Pticairn.

In her book, *Natural Healing for Dogs and Cats*, Diane Stein shows how to use nutrition, minerals, massage, herbs, homeopathy, acupuncture, and psychic healing for the dog's optimal health. She believes that it is the lack of safe, fresh uncontaminated food, water, and air that that decreases a pet's lifespan. I agree with her.

Muffin lived outside, breathing the clean air found in the Cascade Foothills. She drink uncontaminated water from the river, cleaned and purified by nature—the natural ionization process created by the river water tumbling over rocks and purified by the full spectrum light rays from natural sunlight. Most of the time she obtained her own uncontaminated raw meat from the wildlife in the surrounding woods.

The author of *Natural Health for Dogs and Cats* focuses mainly on better nutrition and herbs for dogs and cats.

I found that the far infrared mineral lamp has the same influence and healthful benefits on pets that it does on humans—it provides fast and effective pain relief. Dogs and cats like the heat from the lamp and easily become used to it. The far infrared mineral energy from the lamp is believed to cause the water molecules in the pet's body to vibrate causing a heat reaction using resonant absorption that increases the skin temperature. The end result on animals is the same as it is when used on humans—increased circulation, removal of toxins that interfere with metabolism, and enzyme formation in the activated tissues.

I used this lamp on horses to treat such problems as pulled muscles and ligaments, inflammation, and sores on legs and feet. I found it just as effective on horses as on humans for reducing swelling and pain associated with tissue damage. The number of treatments required will depend on the type and severity of the condition as well as the general health of the horse. Like humans, prolonged use of pain medications require higher and higher doses of medication to achieve the desired pain reduction effect with side effects. Far Infrared Mineral therapy has no side effects in horses!

15

Innovation, Opposition, and Change/Suppression

I was born in Iowa. My mother grew up during the depression and learned the value of hard work to sustain life. During my early childhood years, we lived in a small town and my father was a night watchman. He was quite a bit older than my mother and for several years prior to his death, she supported the family by laundering (clothes). We had electricity in the house, but no running water. The house had a coal furnace and my mother cooked on wood-burning stoves. She started out washing clothes on a washboard. This entailed going outside to a well pump, pumping the water into a pail, hauling the water into the house, and then heating it in a big pan on top of a cooking range. When the water was heated, she would then carry it to the washtub, and repeat the process for the next load of clothes.

She made her own laundry soap from animal fat and lye. She rubbed the dirty clothes against the grooves and rungs in the washboard to clean them. The next step was rinsing them. This she would do by putting the clothes through a hand wringer that was attached to the washtub. She would hold the dripping clothes with one hand and urge them through with the other hand. After rinsing them in cold water, she would then wring them out again and hung them up outside with clothespins on a clothesline. They were dried in this manner in sunshine, sleet, wind, and snow. They froze dry in the wintertime and so did her hands.

When the clothes were dry, she prepared them for ironing. She would sprinkle the clothes that needed to be ironed with water and pack them tightly in an ironing basket. She ironed the clothes with flat irons. She would lay the irons flat on top of the cooking range, and when they were hot, slide them into a device with a handle to hold the hot iron while she transferred it to the ironing board and ironed the clothes. The flat irons were also used in the wintertime at night. Before going to bed she would heat the irons, wrap them in a towel, and place them under the bed covers near the foot of the bed to keep our feet warm. We covered ourselves with quilts made by my mother and other family members. We never threw away a blanket. When it became worn, it was used as a batting in another quilt. Our pillows were made from goose feathers, purchased from a local farmer. Grain sacks were also purchased from the farmers. In those early days, grain was sold in cotton cloth bags. The white sacks were used to make dishtowels and the printed ones were used to make other household items such as pillowcases.

When I was seven years old we moved away from the small town into the rural farming area. This was a little bit like moving back in time. The farmhouse we moved into had no electricity and was heated with a wood stove. There was a cooking range in the kitchen. In the evening, we used kerosene lamps for lighting. Our toilet facilities were located outside and commonly referred to as an outhouse. Sometimes we used torn pages from a magazine or catalog in the place of toilet paper. The outhouse usually had one seat. In the evening and in the wintertime, we used a covered pail as an indoor toilet. Of course, it had to be emptied quite regularly. It was customary to take one bath a week on Saturdays. We used a big, round tub. Water was heated on the stove and carried to the tub. The laundry was performed in the same fashion as before. When family members only bathe once a week, the laundry is not very big either!

A farmer did his shopping on Saturday evening. All of us went to town on Saturday night. The courthouse was built in a square, and the stores were built along the streets adjacent to the courthouse. While the adults shopped, younger children would walk around and around the square. This was a really big event. Farmers would meet neighbors and chat. Children would pair up with other children they knew, and around and around the square they would go. By the time the stores closed at 9:00 p.m., everybody was ready to go home.

My uncle Lawrence liked to spend his Saturday evenings in the saloon. I remember one Saturday night he was arrested for being intoxicated. He tripped and fell down on the saloon floor. Concerned for his welfare, the saloon owner called for the sheriff. When the sheriff came to help him to his car he rebelled because he did not think he was that drunk. The sheriff told him that he was concerned my uncle my get hurt worse the next time he fell. My uncle responded, "I am not drunk, and I did not fall—the floor board flew up and hit me in the face. This story was told at family gatherings for sometime afterwards.

Sunday was a special day. We usually went to church in the morning. Contrary to weekday dinners, dinner was served at noon on the Sabbath, and the meal was usually huge. We usually had fried chicken, mashed potatoes and gravy, and apple pie. Sunday afternoons were spent relaxing, either reading a book or visiting neighbors. Every breakfast was the same—bacon, fried eggs, toast, and corn flakes, served with raw, skimmed milk. During the week, the evening meal was dinner (the bigger meal). Almost every night we had fried potatoes and navy bean soup. The potatoes were always peeled. Most of our bread was homemade white bread. My mother made biscuits quite often. Sometimes it was my responsibility to make the bread. I learned how to knead it by hand and place it in prepared bread pans. We always brushed the top with butter before baking.

Preparing for a meal was a ritual then. I am sorry that my children rarely had the opportunity to experience it. My mother always placed a tablecloth on the table. It was usually my responsibility to set the table. Each person had a place setting of a plate, saucer, cup, and silverware arranged in accordance with that period's etiquette standards. In the summertime fresh cut flowers were always used as a centerpiece. It was customary after the meal to remove the dishes and fold up the tablecloth so it could be used with the next meal. The floor around the table was always swept. The dishes, pots, and pans were always washed (by hand) before retiring for the evening. After the work was all done, it was then time to go to bed.

We always had chickens and lots of eggs. Every spring we would buy little chicks just hatched from the incubator. We used a heat lamp to keep them warm. Some would always die. One of my first jobs after moving to the farm was to clean out the chicken coop with a rake and a pitchfork. The chicken manure was dumped in a pile to be used as a fertilizer when planting the garden and crops. At an early age I learned to cut off a chicken's head with an axe or wring its neck. I learned how to dip the dead chicken in very hot water and then pluck the feathers. When the feathers were removed, I would then remove the bowels and insides, saving the organs such as the gizzard, heart, and liver—they were my favorite pieces. The chicken was then cut, rolled in flour, and fried in lard.

Several times throughout the year, we would butcher a pig. My mother canned the meat—there was a use for almost every part of the pig. Every year we planted a big garden and would eat fresh vegetables from the garden throughout the summer. There were always enough beans, peas, and other vegetables to can for eating during the long wintry months. In addition to the garden, there were always several varieties of apple, peach, and pear trees. My mother made fruit pies, jams, and canned the surplus to be eaten in the wintertime. There were also cherry trees and mulberry trees. What wonderful memories I have!

Housecleaning was a big chore in itself. The floors were usually hardwood with throw rugs. The rugs were taken outside and shaken or beat with a broom, and the floors were swept with a broom. My mother crocheted her own doilies and dresser tops.

After supper dishes were cleaned and put away—it was nice to sit on the front porch in a swing and watch people walk by or just watch the sunset. Today I am amazed that people living in this era would have the time to sit in a swing, relax, and enjoy the crickets singing or watch the firebugs.

As I grew older everything changed. The tractor replaced the horses, television replaced relaxing in the porch swing in the evening, and big corporate farms replaced the small farmer. Chemical fertilizers and pesticides replaced the chicken manure. Self-reliance and independence was replaced with manufactured products and plastic paper. A few years later the industrial age was replaced by the information handling age we live in now. Astronauts have landed on the moon and live in a space station circling the earth. Technology has exploded. I can sit in my living room and cruise the Internet. I have an automatic dishwasher, washing machine, clothes dryer, refrigerator, and a self-cleaning stove and oven. I have modern conveniences to replace the hard work my mother did. Yet, I do not have time to sit on my porch in the evening and watch the sunset. There have been wonderful strides made in medical technology—heart surgery, brain surgery, liver replacement, kidney replacement, and numerous life saving techniques.

In spite of all of these wonderful advances, some things in Western medicine have remained unchanged throughout the last century—the germ theory, discovered by Louis Pasteur, a renowned scientist (1822–1895) is still the foundation on which the American medical doctor's practice is based. In recent years I have wondered why the medical doctor in America has such a prestigious position—the established authority on health care. Even today, with all the other different philosophies on what causes diseases and how to attain good health, the American Medical Association is still given the recognition and legal acknowledgement of setting the standard in health care. Affordable health care for everyone is a popular topic of discussion within our government as the search continues to find a way to provide it without bankrupting the country. There are many voices suggesting alternatives to costly drugs and surgeries but these voices are suppressed, discounted, and/or eliminated from being heard.

In an effort to understand the American health culture and the powerful and influential control the American Medical Association and the pharmaceutical industry have in politics, our health care system, and in the American patient's trust, I conducted my own research of the beginning of health care in the United States. I believe the acceptance of Pasteur's germ theory spawned the lucrative, powerful, and influential pharmaceutical industry and the American Medical

Association, a combination of power commonly referred to as the "opposition" or "establishment." Pasteur and another great scientist by the name of Bechamp lived in the same era—in fact they knew each other. They had different ideas on why people became sick. Pasteur theorized that organisms entering the body from the outside cause disease—Bechamp theorized that it was the environment within the human body that caused diseases (pleomorphism). Bechamp believed that humans were symbiotic partners with a fungus, and when the terrain in the human body changed, the organism changed to survive. When the organism changed from its primitive, harmless form to a mutated form, disease developed. He called these microorganisms "microzyma." He believed the microzyma remained even after the human expired because he found them in calcareous rock and therefore believed that possibly life originates from ashes and dust particles. He believed they were the third element in the blood and played a major role in blood clotting. The scientific community rejected Bechamp's theory, and he died broken-hearted.

Based on the discoveries in the twentieth century by German and American scientists, it looks like the germ theory prevailed more by consensus of opinion among the scientists rather than on scientific discovery. The story is told that Pasteur, on his deathbed, acknowledged that Bechamp was right—it was the terrain! But it was too late!

Nancy Tomes wrote an interesting book, *The Gospel of Germs: Men, Women, and the Microbe in American Life*, and portrays how deep the microbe became imbedded in our culture and penetrated the homes, lives, and consciousness of Americans. The author shows how the germ theory placed a heavy cleaning burden on women, gave birth to the prestigious differentiation in the medical field of the rich, native-born, white male from the poor, non-white, female, and foreign-born medical practitioner, and gave birth to inclusiveness and social reform in the health care industry. This controversial germ theory was eventually accepted as science by the American medical establishment and they have succeeded in keeping lay people ignorant of the true nature of the germ. In spite of all the scientific discoveries of latter-day scientists proving this theory wrong, the "medical establishment" in America has refused to dethrone the germ theory.

At the turn of the century, health care in rural America was comprised of regular medical doctors and medical doctors who developed their own ideas about health and illness. There was also an assortment of other professionals including magnetic healers, bone setters, etc. The public and law gave each professional equal respect and privileges.

As a result of the Flexnor Report in 1910, which characterized the medical colleges as lacking in the integration of science into treatment methods and training, new licensing laws were developed, and a medical profession developed, characterized by white, upper class males. The standards for entrance and training in medical schools increased and the medical doctor's expertise and knowledge grew significantly, public health and sanitation became better, and morbidity rates decreased, raising the public's respect for physicians and helped them become more powerful and controlling. Because of this high status and control, medical doctors can set the boundaries of medical practice and set the function standards for other health care workers. The enhancement of the medical profession gave birth to the medical authority, the American Medical Association, (AMA), who acquired almost a medical education monopoly as a result of the new licensing laws. They were able to eliminate medical competition.

Some stories claim that the AMA initiated attacks on non-allopathic physicians to eliminate them as threats to their authority. By standardizing educational training and professional licensing, allopathic medicine gained authority and control of medicine and established a legal monopoly over the profession (meaning doctors are protected from outside evaluation, free to regulate their own performance and at the same time able to control other health occupations).

In 1895 an innovative magnetic healer named Daniel David Palmer performed his first adjustment in Davenport, Iowa focusing on the nervous system, the spinal column, and the muscles and tendons supporting it. The first patient had been partially deaf for seventeen years and upon examining his spine, Dr. Palmer discovered a lump—he repositioned the vertebra with a gentle thrust and most of Mr. Lillard's hearing was restored—a new approach to healing was born. In 1897, the Palmer School of Chiropractic was opened in Davenport, Iowa.

This new approach to healing emphasized the human body's self-healing abilities and rejected the use of drugs and surgery (anti-germ theory). The chiropractic philosophy is that we are subject to natural laws created by our source (Universal Intelligence or God) and are born with innate intelligence (our connection with our source), which will promote self-healing when not obstructed. This innate intelligence (energy) flows through our body via the brain, spinal cord, and nerves to all tissues of the body. The founding principles of chiropractic state disease is due to toxicity, negative thoughts, and lack of rest and exercise (not from germs that have entered the body from the outside). A spinal bone misalignment can create physical stress on the spinal tissues or nerves causing obstruction of the flow of energy (innate intelligence) from the brain.

As the miracle story was repeated, it stirred up the opposition" and an organized effort was initiated to discredit and eliminate this new healing technique
that challenged the germ theory. An example of this opposition that is still in
operation today can be found in the foreword of my first book, *Breast Cancer:
Death Call or Enlightenment,* written by Dr. Leo J. Bolles, Bellevue, WA.

Because some chiropractors were trying to incorporate medical and other
alternative healing practices into chiropractic, B.J. Palmer fought to get licensure
laws. B.J. Palmer's son, Bartlett J. Palmer, took over the leadership of the chiropractic college. He was a well-known promoter, supposed to have entertained
high government figures in his home and owned several radio stations. The opposition tried to discredit and destroy this new, anti-drug, anti-surgery profession—chiropractors were arrested for practicing without a medical license.
Chiropractic did survive and today is a flourishing alternative for those desiring
not to be treated with drugs or surgery.

I found a story about the rise and fall of another innovative American scientist
named Royal Rife. He did not survive the opposition! In the early 1930s, it is
believed by many that he made an innovative discovery that would have ended all
diseases—he identified the human cancer virus using the world's most powerful
microscope which he had created and called the "Universal Microscope." He
developed a frequency wave device that used a variable frequency, pulsed radio
transmitter to produce a special wave capable of coupling its energy to the human
body. Exposing the disease microorganisms to their own electromagnetic pattern
of oscillation, he was able to destroy them. He developed many new and innovative devices, some of which are still used today and confirmed Bechamp's theory
of pleomorphism!

Royal Rife's technologies would have provided a cure for all diseases and
financially destroyed "the opposition." Using suppression, theft, and arson, his
research papers, equipment (including the world's most powerful microscope),
and laboratory were destroyed. Financially and emotionally broke, the story ends
with Rife becoming an alcoholic and leaving this world in a questionable manner.
His discoveries and accomplishments have been kept alive through a book written by Barry Lynes, entitled *The Rife Report, The Cancer Cure That Worked, Fifty
Years of Suppression.* I checked Amazon.com and could not pull up the book, but
it is my understanding the book can be purchased on other web sites. However,
there is the twenty-first century sequel to it by Barry Lynes, entitled *The Cancer
Conspiracy: Betrayal, Collusion and the Suppression of Alternative Cancer Treatments.*

During the same era, an innovative herbalist by the name of Jethro Kloss (1863–1946) successfully treated cancer patients with the removal of the malignant tumor, a detoxification process, change of diet, herbs, massage, and other natural modalities (a holistic healing approach supporting pleomorphism). He tried to share his cancer cure with medical science and just as they were ready to explore his techniques," the opposition" overshadowed his technologies with the introduction of new miracle drugs that looked promising as a quick cure for cancer and other degenerative diseases. His healing techniques were successfully suppressed and soon forgotten by the medical community. The herbalist left the world a book entitled, *Back to Eden*, in which he shares his knowledge of diseases, herbal remedies, and compassionate love for the human race. I use the book regularly and bought each of my five daughters a copy for Christmas. When I developed a malignant breast tumor several years ago, I looked for a physician who used similar cancer therapies as Jethro Kloss.

About the same time that Rife was researching the cancer virus in America, Professor Gunther Enderlein, a microbiologist in Germany was discovering similar information. He proved that blood was not sterile, and that a microorganism can appear in various stages of development and in various forms without the loss of its specific characteristics. The professor discovered and identified a harmless organism that lives and coexists peacefully within the human body in its basic or primitive form, which he named the Endobiont. The human provides a host body for them and they provide the human with blood platelets. The Endobiont (a fungus) is our symbiotic partner—we cannot live without them. He identified two different species of the mold that he named Asperigillus niger and Mucor racemosus as the cause of many human diseases.

Supposedly the harmless spore form of the mold lives in the human blood where it is believed to assist in the blood clotting process. This scientist developed the Sanum Remedies, which reverts the fungus back to its primitive state after it has mutated and caused cancer from acidosis of the blood. Dr. Enderlein believed that relieving stress, a healthy diet, and the introduction of the primitive form in the body through the Sanum Remedies could cure cancer.

Gaston Naessens, a Quebec biologist, was innovative and developed a dark field microscope (reflects light off tiny organisms (somatids) at angles allowing them to be seen alive that he called the somatiscope. He like, Bechamp and others, believed the somatid mutates when the human immune system becomes weak. Naessens believed somatids to be living organisms dissimilar from bacteria and viruses and described two life cycles—a microcycle with three forms observed in healthy people and a macrocyle consisting of sixteen forms observed in people with degenerative diseases. He believed that in different stages of the cycle, soma-tids may resemble bacteria, yeasts, or fungi and that he can diagnose diseases by observing the number and forms of somatids in the blood. He is purported to believe that when the somatids are exposed to trauma such as pollution or radia-tion they enter an uncontrolled growth cycle that leads to cancer.

He developed the 714X (a mixture of nitrogen and camphor), a cancer ther-apy that strengthens the immune system by returning the somatids to a normal state. He was accused of murder and arrested when one of his patients who had refused traditional cancer therapies died from his treatment. He was vindicated of the charge and his formula accepted as an experimental drug in Canada.

How much longer can the pharmaceutical industry in American hang onto the germ theory? Some people predict that in twenty years the symptom-relieving drug therapy will be replaced by energy medicine and far infrared mineral ther-apy.

16

Alternative Therapies

Today there is an explosion of alternative healing philosophies. Chiropractic has evolved to network chiropractic using network spinal analysis, which is a combination of New Age, Ayurvedic, chiropractic, and other sciences. Network spinal analysis utilizes light touch instead of the old bone crunching techniques to teach the brain new strategies so people can experience the world more fully, adapt to stress, remove tension from the spine and nervous system, and connect with their body's own natural rhythms. This is my choice of health care at the present time and an alternative to drugs and surgery.

Ayurvedic is another increasingly popular therapy in the United States because it addresses three elementary concepts—contact with nature, holism, and diet—and is practiced by Deepok Chopra, M.D., a Western-educated Indian physician who turned to Ayurvedic medicine after converting to the TM religion. It is a holistic system of healing that originated among the Brahmin sages of ancient India 3000-5000 years ago. It is practiced by millions of people all over the world as it embraces the concepts of preventive health care by helping an individual discover a personal knowledge of living. Ayurveda, translated to English, means a systematic art and science approach to living, utilizing all that nature provides such as foods, spices, herbal medicines, colors, metals, massage, and sound to continually strengthen the body and overcome illness.

Ayurvedic medicine is Indian (Eastern) folk medicine and is promoted in American by disciples of Maharishi Mahesh Yogi, the transcendental meditation TM guru. This alternative health therapy focuses on establishing and maintaining the balance of life energies within the human body rather than focusing on individual symptoms. Both Traditional Chinese Medicine and Network Chiropractic embrace similar concepts.

It addresses the uniqueness of each individual. Two people may appear to have similar symptoms, but their life energy may be different and require different remedies. Ayurveda, like network chiropractic, recognizes that all intelligence and wisdom flow from one universal source. It promotes harmony between a person and nature by living a balanced life. It embraces basic universal energies that regulate all natural processes—Tridosha. It seeks to heal the separation and disarray of the mind-body complex and replenish wholeness and harmony to all people. Natural means of disease prevention include herbs, oils, minerals, heat, water, massage, yoga, meditation, and various forms of counseling.

In 1997, the National Institute of Health officially recognized acupuncture as an effective treatment for pain. Acupuncturists are licensed in about thirty-one states and work as independent providers of health care ranging from pain management to women's health problems.

A chiropractor, George G. Goodheart, from Detroit, Michigan, developed Applied Kinesiology (AK) in the 1960s. It is based on the theory that an organ dysfunction is accompanied by a specific muscle weakness. Diseases are diagnosed through muscle-testing procedures and then treated with techniques that include nutritional counseling, acupressure, and exercise. AK uses the principles of functional neurology, anatomy, physiology, biomechanics, biochemistry, Chinese medicine, acupuncture, and massage. Dr. Goodheart discovered that each large muscle relates to a body organ and that a weakness in a muscle could mean that there is a problem in the associated organ. By making the muscle strong again, he was able to improve the function of the organ.

AK is used a lot to test food supplements. If the muscle tested strong, it was a good food supplement for the person—if the muscle remained weak, it was not. He felt that the muscles were indicators of disharmony. Unlike acupuncture, AK is not to be used for emergency medicine, as an AK practitioner is not used to cure cancer and other degenerative diseases. It is used as a holistic approach to preventive medicine, restoring normal nerve function, achieving normal endocrine and other internal organ functions, and to restore postural balance and range of motion.

Bioenergetics is a therapy that I have always had a hard time understanding exactly what it is. I know that it is a bodywork approach. It is a form of therapy based on the teachings of Wilhelm Reich, who worked under Sigmund Freud in the early part of the twentieth century, linking physical pain, muscle tension, and postural disorders with the state of mind. It demonstrates that suppressed emotions, unhappiness, and anger can block energy-flow and cause physical distress. It focuses on the pattern of muscular tension and how the tension relates to the person's emotional history and childhood relationships.

Reich broke away from Freud when he discovered that the whole body, not just the mind, is an indicator of a person's mental and emotional health. When learning about bioenergetics, I realized that this philosophy is incorporated into many other therapies, including network chiropractic. Both of these techniques entail working with the mind and body to enable the release of tension derived through social conditioning that restricts self-expression and lowers self-esteem.

Chelation therapy is where a drug is administered to draw toxic metals from the bloodstream so the body can eliminate them more effectively. Physicians in America have used it since 1950 to treat lead poisoning and other heavy metals.

Colon therapy is a controversial technique in which a colonic is used as part of the detoxification process to eliminate or neutralize toxins in the body. Health professionals are either adamant about the usefulness of a colonic and recommend regular use to stay healthy, or they are completely against it. Often it is used with fasting. Those who endorse the colonics believe that the primary cause of disease is the accumulation of wastes in the colon.

CranioSacral therapy is a technique used to gently manipulate the bones of the skull to enhance the functioning of the Cranio Sacral system. I believe a doctor at Michigan State University developed the technique.

Deep tissue bodywork covers many therapies including Hellerwork and Rolfing. This type of massage goes deeper than the Swedish massage where the therapist applies deep pressure to the muscle tissue to release tension.

Environmental therapy is used to identify chemicals and allergens that may cause illness or allergies in a person's life, home, and work. Once the sensitivities are identified, desensitization of the guilty culprit is initiated. I went through several years of desensitization for both food and environmental sensitivities.

Enzyme therapy is used to improve digestion and eliminate malabsorption problems through enzyme supplementation of essential nutrients. My alternative therapy doctor used this type of therapy when treating me for breast cancer.

Hands of Light healing is a technique taught by Barbara Brennan. It is a four-year program and teaches the therapist to work with the client's energy field.

Homeopathy therapy is the introduction of tiny doses of natural substances that act as a catalyst to get the body to heal itself naturally.

Naturopathic medicine uses natural methods to treat people that might include nutritional supplements, herbs, homeopathy, and other natural modalities. In recent years, naturopathic doctors are licensed as physicians to diagnose and treat in a general family practice in many states.

Neural therapy was developed in Germany and involves the injections of local anesthetics and homeopathic formulas into the nervous system to block the flow of energy. Neural therapy was used on my root canal to block negative energy flow.

Oxygen therapy was developed in Germany and is used to increase the supply of oxygen in the body and includes hydrogen peroxide therapy and ozone therapy.

Polarity therapy is used to balance the flow of energy through the body by gentle touch, diet counseling, and exercise.

Reflexology and foot reflexology is similar to acupressure in which pressure is applied to certain points to stimulate organs and glands.

Reiki is an energy exercise that is used to restore and balance life force energy throughout the body for mental, emotional, spiritual, and physical balancing.

I have only mentioned a few of the alternative therapies available today. I have tried many of the foregoing, and others I just have heard of or know someone else who has tried them. There are so many different energy approaches to better health and so many therapies focusing on the integration of mind and body as an approach to healing such as *Energy Medicine* by David Eden, David Feinstein, Brooks Garden, Illustrator, Caroline Myss,

I believe that pain-free living and increased life longevity can become a lifestyle for many of us through the frequent use of the far infrared mineral lamp, which can provide fast and effective pain relief, increased blood circulation, and increased energy.

Bibliography

Becker, Robert O. Cross Currents: *The Promise of Electromedicine, the Perils of Electropollution*

Becker, R.,Seldon, N. & Bichell, D. *The Body Electric: Electromagnetism and the Foundation of Life.* Morrow, William, & Co. 1987

Batmanghelidj, Fereydoon (Illustrator). *Your Body's Many Cries for Water*

Burr, Harold Saxton. *Blueprint for Immortality: The Electric Patterns of Life*

Cohen, Misha Ruth, Doner, Kalia (Contributory), Michals, Robin (Illustrator). *The Chinese Way to Healing: Many Paths to Wholeness*

Duggan, Sandra. *Edgar Cayce's Guide to Colon Care: The First Step to Vibrant Health*

Epstein, D. & Altman, N. *The Twelve Stages of Healing, A Network Approach to Wholeness.* Amber-Allen Publishing. 1995.

Epstein, D. *Healing Myths, Healing Magic: Breaking the Spell of Old Illusions; Reclaiming our Power to Heal.* Amber-Allen Publishing. 2000.

James L., Ph.D. Oachman, Candance, Ph.D. Pert. *Energy Medicine: The Scientific Basis of Bioenergy Therapies.*

Kloss, J. *Back to Eden.* Revised and Expanded Edition by Promise K. Moffet. Back to Eden Publishing Co. 1990.

Kordich, Jay. *The Juiceman's Power of Juicing*

Lynes, Barry. *The Cancer Conspiracy: Betrayal, Collusion and the Suppression of Alternative Cancer Treatments.*

Ott, John N.*Health and Light: The Effects of Natural and Artificial Light on Man and Other Living Things.*

Pticairn, Richard H. *Natural Health for Dogs and Cats*

Schoonover, Kara Lee. *Breast Cancer: Death Call or Enlightenment*

Stein, Diane. *Natural Healing for Dogs and Cats*

Tomes, Nancy. *The Gospel of Germs: Men, Women, and the Microbe in American Life*

Index

0-595-27263-0